CLIN

THE AACN SYNERGY MODEL

FOR PATIENT CARE

EDITORS

Sonya R. Hardin, PhD, RN, CCRN, APRN
Associate Professor
School of Nursing
Adult Health Nursing Department
University of North Carolina at Charlotte
Charlotte, North Carolina

Roberta Kaplow, PhD, RN, CCNS, CCRN
Clinical Professor
Nell Hodgson Woodruff School of Nursing
Emory University
Atlanta, Georgia

JONES AND BARTLETT PUBLISHERS
Sudbury, Massachusetts
BOSTON   TORONTO   LONDON   SINGAPORE

World Headquarters
Jones and Bartlett Publishers
40 Tall Pine Drive
Sudbury, MA 01776
978-443-5000
info@jbpub.com
www.jbpub.com

Jones and Bartlett Publishers Canada
2406 Nikanna Road
Mississauga, ON L5C 2W6
CANADA

Jones and Bartlett Publishers International
Barb House, Barb Mews
London W6 7PA
UK

Library of Congress Cataloging-in-Publication Data

Synergy for clinical excellence : the AACN synergy model for patient
    care / editors, Sonya R. Hardin, Roberta Kaplow.
    p. ; cm.
  Includes bibliographical references and index.
  ISBN 0-7637-2601-X (pbk.)
    1. Intensive care nursing—Standards. 2. Nursing models. 3. Nurse
and patient. 4. Outcome assessment (Medical care) I. Hardin,
Sonya R. II. Kaplow, Roberta.
  [DNLM: 1. Critical Illness—nursing. 2. Nursing Care—standards.
3. Certification. 4. Models, Nursing. 5. Nurse Practitioners.
6. Treatment Outcome. WY 154 S992 2004]
RT120.I5S97 2004
616.02′8—dc22

                                                            2004007883

Acquisitions Editor: Kevin Sullivan
Production Manager: Amy Rose
Associate Production Editor: Renée Sekerak
Editorial Assistant: Amy Sibley
Marketing Manager: Ed McKenna
Associate Marketing Manager: Emily Ekle
Manufacturing and Inventory Coordinator: Amy Bacus
Composition: Auburn Associates, Inc.
Cover Design: Kristin E. Ohlin
Printing and Binding: Malloy Inc.
Cover Printing: Malloy Inc.

Printed in the United States of America
08 07 06 05   10 9 8 7 6 5 4 3 2

DEDICATION

This book is dedicated to Jack, Eleanor, Susan, Ali, Texas, Pauline, James, and Bria. We are indeed grateful for your love, support, and encouragement during our time away from home working on the production of this book.

CONTENTS

FOREWORD

The AACN Synergy Model for Patient Care rests on a remarkably simple premise: *Optimal outcomes result from the synergy of a nurse's competencies matching the needs of patients and their families.*

The Synergy Model draws from Virginia Henderson's often-quoted definition of nursing:

"The unique function of the nurse is to assist the individual, sick or well, in the performance of those activities contributing to health or its recovery [or to peaceful death] that he would perform unaided if he had the necessary strength, will, or knowledge." (Henderson, page 15)

What began as an effort to develop a conceptual model for specialty certification in critical care has evolved into one of the most widely applicable frameworks for nursing practice.

Today the model is being applied in a wide range of nursing situations. Nursing position descriptions at Children's Hospital in Boston and All Children's Hospital in St. Petersburg, Florida, are based on it. So are the professional advancement program and an innovative patient safety initiative at the 1,200-bed Clarian Health Partners system in Indianapolis, Indiana. Nursing degree programs, including a new online master's in acute care nursing, at Duquesne University in Pittsburgh, Pennsylvania, also will use the model.

With this book, Sonya R. Hardin, Roberta Kaplow, and their collaborating contributors bring the Synergy Model to the attention of many audiences that may choose to apply it. We commend their energy and enthusiasm for making the model accessible to clinicians, advanced practice nurses, educators, managers, administrators, and others who will be captivated by its simple pragmatism.

Dorrie K. Fontaine RN, DNSc, FAAN
President 2003–2004
American Association of Critical-Care Nurses

Suzanne S. Prevost RN, PhD
Chair 2003–2004
AACN Certification Corporation

Virginia A. Henderson. *The Nature of Nursing.* 1966. New York: Macmillan.

PREFACE

This book is a tribute to all the critical care nurses who serve patients worldwide. It is based upon a decade of work by the American Association of Critical-Care Nurses (AACN) in the development of a conceptual framework for certified practice: The Synergy Model. The purpose of this book is to provide nurses with the clinical knowledge needed to apply The AACN Synergy Model in practice and to help prepare nurses for certification examinations offered by AACN. This text can be utilized in a nursing course that focuses on nursing theory and conceptual frameworks.

Chapter 1 presents a brief history of the development of the model and the patient and nurse characteristics inherent in The AACN Synergy Model. Section I serves as a foundation for understanding the application of the concepts in each of the chapters that follow. Section II provides in-depth chapters focusing on each patient characteristic in the model with application to patient situations to further explicate the use of the model in practice. Section III consists of chapters focused on the nurse characteristics with applications to practice. Section IV has sample test questions for those nurses seeking to obtain certification through AACN. These questions provide the nurse with further examples of the integration of the model into practice.

We would like to thank the contributors who have been actively engaged in the recent study of practice conducted by the AACN Certification Corporation in collaboration with Professional Education Services (PES). This book has been developed to enhance the understanding of The AACN Synergy Model and to provide a reference to those who are in the process of utilizing the model in their practice.

Sonya R. Hardin

ACKNOWLEDGMENTS

We gratefully acknowledge the outstanding contributors of this text. Without the expertise of these scholars, this work would not have been possible.

We express sincere appreciation to AACN and the AACN Certification Corporation for permission to use The AACN Synergy Model graphic representation and for their commitment to optimize patient care through certified practice. We would like to recognize Carol Hartigan and Elizabeth Miller for their continued insightfulness in integrating The AACN Synergy Model into certified practice.

We also thank the following people at Jones and Bartlett: Amy Sibley and Penny Glynn.

Lastly, a special thanks must be extended to our families and friends who have supported us during the production of the book. Their support and encouragement has helped to sustain us during the final production.

Sonya R. Hardin
Roberta Kaplow

CONTRIBUTORS

Deborah L. Bingaman, MS, RN, CPNP, CCNS
Pediatric Nurse Practitioner
Pulmonary Hypertension Program
Pediatric Heart Lung Center
The Children's Hospital
Denver, Colorado

Michael W. Day, MSN, RN, CCRN
Outreach Educator/Clinical Nurse
Specialist
North West Medstar
Spokane, Washington

Beth C. Diehl-Svrjcek, MS, RN, CCRN, CCM, NNP, LNCC
NICU/Special Needs Child Care Manager
Johns Hopkins Healthcare, LLC
Baltimore, Maryland

Sonya R. Hardin, PhD, RN, CCRN, APRN
Associate Professor
School of Nursing
Adult Health Nursing Department
University of North Carolina at Charlotte
Charlotte, North Carolina

Roberta Kaplow, PhD, RN, CCNS, CCRN
Clinical Professor
Nell Hodgson Woodruff School of
Nursing
Emory University
Atlanta, Georgia

Marthe J. Moseley, PhD, RN, CCRN, CCNS
Clinical Nurse Specialist, Critical Care
South Texas Veterans Health Care System
Audie L. Murphy Division
San Antonio, Texas

Daphne Stannard, PhD, RN, CCRN, CCNS
Assistant Professor
San Francisco State University
School of Nursing
San Francisco, California

Linda L. Steele, PhD, RN, APRN, BC
Associate Professor
School of Nursing
Adult Health Nursing Department
University of North Carolina at Charlotte
Charlotte, North Carolina

Darla Ura, MA, RN, APRN, BC
Associate Professor
Nell Hodgson Woodruff School of
Nursing
Emory University
Atlanta, Georgia

SECTION I

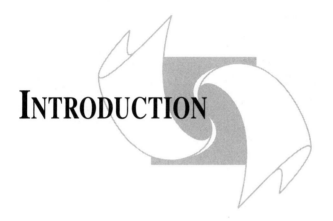

INTRODUCTION

CHAPTER 1

INTRODUCTION TO THE AACN SYNERGY MODEL FOR PATIENT CARE

Sonya R. Hardin, PhD, RN, CCRN, APRN

INTRODUCTION

During the 1990s, the American Association of Critical-Care Nurses (AACN) envisioned a new paradigm for clinical practice. The vision was to transcend the current thinking of practice as a series of tasks to a health care system driven by the needs of patients in which nurses make optimal contributions to patient outcomes. In 1993, the AACN Certification Corporation convened a think tank to develop a conceptual framework for certified practice. The think tank included nationally recognized experts, including Martha A. Q. Curley, Mairead Hickey, Patricia Hooper, Wanda Johanson, Bonnie Niebuhr, Sarah Sanford, and Gayle Whitman. Members of the think tank believed that certified practice is more than a series of tasks and should be grounded in nurses meeting the needs of patients and influencing optimal outcomes (Curley, 1998).

At the time, the idea seemed quite radical because certification in critical care was awarded on the basis of hours worked in a critical care setting, the number and type of tasks performed, and an examination based on body systems. Introduction of the proposed conceptual framework at the AACN National Teaching Institute (NTI) in 1994 prompted nurses to question the soundness of using a conceptual model based on patient and nurse characteristics. During a meeting of AACN members there was difficulty seeing the value of redefining nurses' practice into more than the sum of its parts.

During the 1994 NTI, the AACN Certification Corporation board of directors articulated the importance of linking certified practice with patient outcomes. Of great importance was the ability to articulate nurses' unique contribution in caring for critically ill patients regardless of where the care is delivered. The think tanks described 13 patient needs and 9 characteristics of nurses. The patient characteristics included compensation, resiliency, margin of error, predictability, complexity, vulnerability, physiological stability, risk of death, independence, self-determination, involvement in care decisions, engagement, and resource availability. These characteristics are based on universal needs of the patients. In order to meet specific patient needs, nurses require certain characteristics. The think tank identified 9 characteristics of nurses: engagement, skilled clinical practice, agency, caring practices, system management, team work, diversity responsiveness, experiential learning, and innovator-evaluator. The synergy emerging from the interaction between the patient needs and the nurse characteristics results in optimum outcomes for the patient. The think tank members believed that these characteristics of the nurse would determine competencies for certified practice (Caterinicchio, 1995). A synergistic nature should exist between the patient and the nurse. If correctly matched, this mutuality ensures that patient needs are met.

In 1995, the AACN Certification Corporation board of directors appointed a group of subject matter experts from across the United States to refine the conceptual model and guide a study of practice and job analysis of critical care nurses. Professional Examination Services (PES) was retained to work with this group to refine the model and to test the validity of the concepts in critical care practice. The study would serve as the basis for a revised certification exam. The subject matter experts were Martha A. Q. Curley, Duanne Foster-Smith, Deborah Gloskey, Janet Fraser Hale, Teresa Halloran, Sonya R. Hardin, Patricia Hooper, Mairead Hickey, Vickie Keough, Patricia Moloney-Harmon, Kathleen Shurpin, and Daphne Stannard. This group refined the patient and nurse characteristics as well as delineated a continuum for the characteristics. The patient characteristics were distilled from the original 13 patient needs into the following 8 concepts:

1. resiliency
2. vulnerability
3. stability
4. complexity
5. resource availability
6. participation in care
7. participation in decision making
8. predictability

The nurse characteristics were also merged into 8 concepts:

1. clinical judgment
2. advocacy
3. caring practices
4. collaboration
5. systems thinking
6. response to diversity
7. clinical inquiry
8. facilitation of learning (AACN Certification Corporation, 2003a)

According to the model, each patient brings a unique set of characteristics to the health care situation. Among the many characteristics that are present, 8 are consistently seen in patients who experience critical events. These 8 characteristics are consistently assessed by nurses in variable levels given each patient situation. These characteristics, as well as other patterns that are unique to each patient's circumstances, should be assessed in every patient.

Resiliency is the patient's capacity to return to a restorative level of functioning using a compensatory coping mechanism. The level of resiliency assessed in patients is often dependent upon their ability to rebound after an insult. This ability can be influenced by many factors including age, comorbidities, and compensatory mechanisms that are intact.

Vulnerability is the level of susceptibility to actual or potential stressors that may adversely affect patient outcomes. Vulnerability can be impacted by the patient's physiological make-up or health behaviors exhibited by the patient.

Stability refers to the patient's ability to maintain a steady state of equilibrium. Response to therapies and nursing interventions can impact the stability of the patient.

Complexity is the intricate entanglement of two or more systems. Systems refer to either physiological or emotional states of the body, family dynamics, or environmental interactions with the patient. The more systems involved, the more complex are the patterns displayed by the patient.

Resource availability is influenced by the extent of resources brought to the situation by the patient, family, and community. The resources can present as technical, fiscal, personal, psychological, social, or supportive in nature. The more resources that a person brings to the health care situation, the greater the potential for a positive outcome.

Participation in care is the participation by a patient and family in being engaged in the delivery of care. Patient and family participation can be influenced by educational background, resource availability, and cultural background.

Participation in decision making is the level of engagement of the patient and family in comprehending the information provided by health care providers and acting upon this information to execute informed decisions. Patient and family engagement in clinical decisions can be impacted by the knowledge level of the patient, his or her capacity to make decisions given the insult, the cultural background (i.e., beliefs and values), and the level of inner strength during a crisis (AACN Certification Corporation, 2003a).

Predictability is the characteristic that allows one to expect a certain course of events or course of illness.

The nurse characteristics can be considered competencies that are essential for those providing care to the critically ill. The nursing competencies were validated in 1997 by a study of practice and job analysis conducted by the Professional Examination Services (PES) on behalf of the AACN Certification Corporation. PES mailed the patient characteristics, along with the varying levels of patient acuity, to nurses and asked the nurses to rate each profile indicating the perceived level of criticality of the patient given the leveling of the characteristic. All 8 competencies reflect an integration of knowledge, skills, and experience of the nurse.

Clinical judgment is the clinical reasoning utilized by a health care provider in the delivery of care. It consists of critical thinking and nursing skills that are acquired through a process of integrating education, experiential knowledge, and evidence-based guidelines. The integration of knowledge brings about the clinical decisions made during the course of care provided to the patient.

Advocacy is working on another's behalf when the other is not capable of advocating for him- or herself. The nurse serves as a moral agent in identifying and helping to resolve ethical and clinical concerns within the clinical setting.

Pt c̄ PICC line wanted to place central for CVP

Caring practices are the constellation of nursing interventions that create a compassionate, supportive, and therapeutic environment for patients and staff, with the aim of promoting comfort and healing and preventing unnecessary suffering. Caring behaviors include compassion, vigilance, engagement, and responsiveness to the patient and family.

Collaboration is the nurse working with others to promote optimal outcomes. The patient, family, and members of various health care disciplines work toward promoting optimal and realistic patient goals.

Systems thinking comprises the tools and knowledge that the nurse utilizes to recognize the interconnected nature within and across the health care or non-health care system. The ability to understand how one decision can impact the whole is integral to systems thinking. The nurse uses a global perspective in clinical decision making and has the ability to negotiate the needs of the patient and family through the health care system.

Response to diversity is the sensitivity to recognize, appreciate, and incorporate differences into the provision of care. Nurses need to recognize the individuality of each patient while observing for patterns that respond to nursing interventions. Individuality can be observed in the patient's spiritual beliefs, ethnicity, family configuration, lifestyle values, and use of alternative and complementary therapies.

Clinical inquiry is the ongoing process of questioning and evaluating practice, providing informed practice, and innovating through research and experiential learning. Clinical inquiry evolves as the nurse moves from novice to expert. At the expert level, the nurse improves, deviates, and/or individualizes standards and guidelines to meet the needs of the patient.

Facilitation of learning means that the nurse facilitates learning for patients, families, nursing staff, physicians and other health care disciplines, and community through both formal and informal facilitation of learning. Education should be provided based on individual strengths and weaknesses of the patient and family. The educational level of the patient should be considered in the design of the plan of educating the patient and family to ensure informed decisions. Creative methods should be developed to ensure patient and family comprehension.

Each nurse and patient characteristic is understood on a continuum from one to five. The level of each patient characteristic is critical in the competency required of the nurse (AACN Certification Corporation, 2003a). The levels of each characteristic are discussed in the following chapters of this text.

The AACN Synergy Model for Patient Care (Figure 1–1) is based on five assumptions (AACN, 2000, p. 55):

1. Patients are biological, social, and spiritual entities who are present at a particular developmental stage. The whole patient (body, mind, and spirit) must be considered.
2. The patient, family, and community all contribute to providing a context for the nurse-patient relationship.
3. Patients can be described by a number of characteristics. Characteristics are connected and contribute to each other. Characteristics cannot be looked at in isolation.
4. Nurses can be described on a number of dimensions. The interrelated dimensions paint a profile of the nurse.

Figure 1–1

The Synergy Model delineates three levels of outcomes: those derived from the patient, those derived from the nurse, and those derived from the healthcare system.

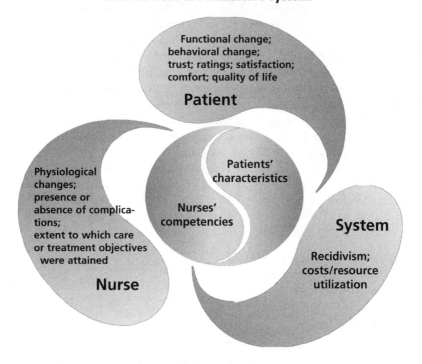

From "Patient-Nurse Synergy: Optimizing Patients' Outcomes"
By Martha AQ Curley, RN, PhD, CCRN
American Journal of Critical Care, January 1998, Volume 7, No. 1, Page 69

5. A goal of nursing is to restore a patient to an optimal level of wellness as defined by the patient. Death can be an acceptable outcome in which the goal of nursing care is to move a patient toward a peaceful death.

In 2002, a practice analysis task force appointed by the AACN Certification Corporation expanded the assumptions of the model to include the following (AACN Certification Corporation, 2003b; Muenzen et al., 2004):

- The nurse creates the environment for the care of the patient. The context/ environment of care also affects what the nurse can do.
- There is an interrelatedness between impact areas. The nature of the inter-relatedness may change as the function of experience, situation, and setting changes.
- The nurse may work to optimize outcomes for patients, families, health care providers, and the health care system/organization.
- The nurse brings his or her background to each situation, including various levels of education/knowledge and skills/experience.

These assumptions underlay the conceptual framework and establish the context for understanding the Synergy Model. The purpose of nursing is to meet the needs of patients and families and to provide safe passage through the health care system during a time of crisis. The Synergy Model is a conceptual framework for designing practice and developing the competencies required to care for critically ill patients. Even though the Synergy Model is used as a blueprint for certified practice, the model has far reaching implications for the practice of nursing and other health care professions. The model could be utilized to develop nursing curriculums and for conducting research focused on the interrelationship of competencies and patient outcomes.

According to the Synergy Model, when patient characteristics and nurse competencies match, patient outcomes are optimized. In 1996, the AACN Certification Corporation appointed a new think tank to articulate optimal outcomes. Members of this think tank included Patricia Benner, Melissa Biel, Martha A. Q. Curley, Wanda Johanson, Marion Johnson, Marguerite Kinney, Benton Lutz, Patricia Moloney-Harmon, Alvin Tarlov, and Cheri White. Outcomes are considered patient conditions measured along a continuum (Curley, 1998). The task force identified six major quality outcome indicators:

1. patient and family satisfaction
2. rate of adverse incidents
3. complication rate
4. adherence to the discharge plan
5. mortality rate
6. the patient's length of stay

The AACN Synergy Model was found to be congruent with outcomes derived from the patient, nurse, and health care system. Outcomes derived from the patient include functional changes, behavioral changes, trust, satisfaction, comfort, and quality of life. Outcomes derived from nursing competencies include physiological changes, the presence or absence of complications, and the extent treatment objectives were obtained (Curley, 1998). Outcome data derived from the health care system include readmission rates, length of stay, and cost utilization per case.

The 2002 practice analysis task force members were Patricia Atkins, Deborah Becker, Deborah Bingaman, Nancy Blake, Jo Ellen Craghead, Beth Diehl-Svrjcek, Sonya R. Hardin, Melissa Hutchinson, Linda Jackson, Roberta Kaplow, Marthe Moseley, Marlene Roman, Daphne Stannard, Karen Thomason, and Darla Ura. They were charged to work with PES in conducting an updated study of practice and job analysis. These individuals, with facilitation from PES, undertook a 2-year study for the purpose of reviewing and enhancing the nurse characteristics so as to be reflective of the practice of entry-level critical care nurses, CCRN-certified nurses, and advanced practice critical care nurses. The nurse characteristics were further delineated and expanded through the development of descriptive behaviors for entry-level, competent, and expert critical care nurses as well as descriptors for the nurse practitioner and clinical nurse specialist. PES conducted focus panels, critical incident interviews, and subject matter expert interviews of the delineated descriptors for the nurse characteristics. After these data were collected and presented to the task force, further revisions occurred and these revisions were submitted as a survey to entry-level critical care nurses, CCRN-certified nurses, and advanced practice critical care nurses. The findings from these surveys indicated a difference in the level of nurse characteristic between entry-level critical care nurses, CCRN- and CCNS-certified nurses, and acute care nurse practitioners. These distinct differences will be integrated into the future examinations offered by the AACN Certification Corporation.

Research is needed to further validate the link between outcome criteria and certified practice. Funding needs to be focused on collecting data of patient, nurse, and system outcomes in units that have a high percentage of certified nurses as compared to similar institutions that do not have a high number of certified nurses. These data could help to revise and validate the model. The AACN Synergy Model currently serves as the framework for the CCRN, CCNS, and PCCN (progressive care) exams offered by the AACN Certification Corporation.

REFERENCES

AACN Certification Corporation. (2003a). *The AACN Synergy Model for Patient Care*. Available at: http://www.aacn.org/certcorp/certcorp.nsf/vwdoc/Syn Model?opendocument. Accessed May 11, 2004.

AACN Certification Corporation. (2003b). *CCRN—Certification for Adult, Pediatric and Neonatal Critical Care Nurses* [CCRN Job Analysis]. Available at: http://www.certcorp.org/certcorp.nsf/certcerp.ccrn. Accessed May 11, 2004.

American Association of Critical-Care Nurses. (2000). *Standards for Acute and Critical Care Nursing Practice*, (3rd ed.). Aliso Viejo, CA: AACN Critical Care Publications.

Caterinicchio, M. (for the AACN Certification Corporation). (1995). Redefining Nursing According to Patients' and Families' Needs: An Evolving Concept. *AACN Clinical Issues* 6(1): 153–156.

Curley, M. A. Q. (1998). Patient-Nurse Synergy: Optimizing Patients' Outcomes. *American Journal of Critical Care* 7(1): 64–72.

Muenzen, P. M., Greenberg, S., and Pirrol, K. A. (2004). *Final Report of a Comprehensive Study of Critical Care Nursing Practice.* Available at: http://www.certcorp.org/certcorp.nsf/certcerp.ccrn.

SECTION II

PATIENT CHARACTERISTICS

CHAPTER 2

RESILIENCY

Roberta Kaplow, PhD, RN, CCNS, CCRN

INTRODUCTION

Why are some people able to react to difficult situations with less severe consequences than others exposed to the same events (Humphreys, 2003)? Why do some people see the future as bleak with barriers perceived as brick walls while others see these adversities as surmountable? Some people have the ability to bounce back, whatever comes their way (Lauer, 2002). Why do some patients recover nicely after illness and handle life without too much disturbance to their quality of life despite some adversity (Talsma, 1995)? This is resiliency.

Resiliency has been defined as the ability to achieve, retain, or regain a level of physical or emotional health after a devastating illness or loss (Felten and Hall, 2001). Resiliency has been studied in relation to several diverse untoward events and atrocities. Some of these include the Holocaust, famine, environmental conditions, battered women, breast cancer, HIV/AIDS, and other diseases with high levels of associated morbidity and mortality.

Research on resiliency has increased significantly over the past several decades (Miller and MacIntosh, 1999). It has been described by assessing people confronted with difficult conditions and how they were able to cope (Greene, 2002). A number of theories of resiliency exist. Two of these include "an acceptance of reality, a deep belief that life is meaningful" and "an uncanny ability to improvise" (Lauer, 2002, p. 29).

It is essential to understand what factors promote or enhance a patient's resiliency (Woodgate, 1999). Theories have been suggested regarding the relationship between resiliency and other factors. Relationships have been reported with spirituality and social support. These factors contributed to levels of resiliency in patients with HIV disease (Poblete, 2000). Other significant factors associated with resiliency include faith, hope, having a living relative, and having memories of one's roots (Lothe and Heggen, 2003). Factors identified in older women that enhance resiliency include determination, previous experience with hardship, access to care, culturally based health beliefs, family support, self-care activities, and caring for others (Felten and Hall, 2001; Felten, 2001).

One of the other factors that has been associated with an individual's level of resiliency is the quality of resources the individual has to help with the adjustment to an adverse situation. These may include an individual's own resources, family, and community. On any given day or time, any or all of these resources can be used to deal with stress (Callahan, 2003).

In one study of people aged 75 and older, females and older subjects had lower levels of resiliency. This was attributed to being less involved in physical activity, exercise, and community. Marital status and a higher social status had a weak correlation with resiliency in this study (Talsma, 1995).

Evaluation of resilient people revealed that they have a sober, practical view of aspects of reality that are consistent with survival. Another facet of resiliency reported is a "search for meaning"; that is, many individuals can find some meaning in adverse circumstances (Lauer, 2002).

Why is resiliency important? Sequela of resiliency has been reported. These include avoidance of distress and successful ability to cope and function (Tusaie-Mumford, 2001). Use of a resiliency scale revealed a positive relationship between resiliency and physical health, morale, and life satisfaction, and a negative relationship with depression. That is, people with higher levels of resiliency were less likely to have feelings of depression (Wagnild and Young, 1993).

In a study with children, it was found that those with high levels of resiliency had good temperaments, were easy to get along with, had an intact support system and self-esteem, and were in good physical health. Data from that same study revealed factors that had a negative impact on resiliency, including poverty and prolonged absence of a parental unit (Werner and Smith, 1992).

DEFINITION

The AACN Synergy Model definition of resiliency is "the patient's capacity to return to a restorative level of functioning by using compensatory and coping mechanisms" (Curley, 1998). According to the AACN, patients with low levels of resiliency (Level 1) are those unable to mount a response, those with failure of compensatory/coping mechanisms, minimal reserves, and brittle. A Level 3 patient is considered moderately resilient. These patients are able to mount a moderate response, to initiate some degree of compensation, and to have moderate reserves. A Level 5 patient is considered highly resilient. This individual is able to mount and maintain a response, and has intact compensatory mechanisms, strong reserves, and endurance (AACN, 2003). A highly resilient individual is able to cultivate strength to potentially meet challenging situations or conditions. Resiliency connotes that the individual has adapted to other stressors in the past. Data support that each individual "has an innate capacity for resiliency" (Resiliency in Action, Inc. © 2002, 2003).

Mr. J is a 56-year-old patient diagnosed with non-Hodgkin's lymphoma. His past medical history is significant for myocardial infarction 5 years ago, borderline renal insufficiency, and gout. He was admitted to the hospital for prechemotherapy hydration and treatment of his disease. He received hydration for 48 hours with urinary alkalinization with 100 mEq of sodium bicarbonate/liter of intravenous fluids during that time. The day following initiation of chemotherapy, Mr. J's labs are as follows:

Na	135
K	6.8
Cl	102
CO_2	22
Glucose	126
BUN	30
Creat	1.2
Phos	10
Ca	7.2
Uric Acid	11.2

Mr. J was diagnosed with acute tumor lysis syndrome and he was transferred to the intensive care unit for management of metabolic imbalances and cardiac monitoring. Upon admission, the nurses noted ST segment elevation, consistent with hyperkalemia. Admission orders included 10 units of regular insulin and 25 grams of $D_{50}W$ IV push, aluminum hydroxide 30cc every 4 hours, allopurinol 300 mg daily, and forced diuresis with furosemide (Lasix®). Eight hours later his labs were as follows:

Na	139
K	5.2
Cl	104
CO_2	21
Glucose	153
BUN	27
Creat	1.0
Phos	9.2
Ca	7.4
Uric Acid	10.4

After 3 days, Mr. J's electrolytes were normalized and he was discharged from the intensive care unit. He tolerated the rest of his therapy and was discharged from the hospital several days later.

APPLICATION OF THE CASE STUDY TO THE SYNERGY MODEL

Acute tumor lysis syndrome (ATLS) is a life-threatening oncologic emergency characterized by electrolyte imbalances and metabolic derangements that can lead to renal failure and multiple organ dysfunction syndrome. It is characterized by hyperkalemia, hyperphosphatemia, hyperuricemia, and hypocalcemia. These electrolyte abnormalities result when antineoplastic therapy kills cancer cells. The killed (or lysed) cells release their intracellular components into the patient's bloodstream. Mr. J had a number of risk factors identified by the nursing staff for the development of ATLS, specifically renal insufficiency, non-Hodgkin's lymphoma, and gout. Renal insufficiency is a risk factor because of the decreased ability of the kidneys to excrete the excess potassium and phosphorus that gets displaced from the intracellular compartment of cancer and normal cells with the induction of antineoplastic therapy. Nucleic acids similarly get displaced from the intracellular compartment and are converted to uric acid by the liver. Uric acid crystals form in the ureters and distal convoluted tubules. Gout is a risk factor because of the excess uric acid present with that condition (Doane, 2002; Gobel, 2002; Kaplow, 2002).

Despite receiving vigorous hydration and urinary alkalinization, Mr. J developed this oncologic emergency. His life-threatening metabolic derangements made him a candidate for admission to the intensive care unit. Early recognition and prompt aggressive interventions for the syndrome enhanced Mr. J's resiliency. He was able to rebound from several potentially fatal metabolic imbalances. Consistent with the AACN Synergy Model, Mr. J is a Level 5, highly resilient. He demonstrated resiliency by being able to bounce back from and successfully adapt to an adverse clinical condition.

Had the nursing staff not identified Mr. J as being at risk, his clinical course might have turned out differently. The nursing staff was conscientious with following up and recognizing the need for allopurinol (Zyloprim®) based on Mr. J's uric acid levels, monitoring for the development of acute uric acid nephropathy, and preventing acute renal failure from uric acid crystals formation. Continuing aggressive fluid intake, urinary alkalinization, and forced diuresis helped avert formation of calcium-phosphorus precipitate. Lack of assessment and prompt management of hyperkalemia could have resulted in cardiac arrest. This latter scenario, if left unrecognized and untreated, would have resulted in death. In this circumstance, according to the tenets of the AACN Synergy Model, Mr. J's level of resiliency would have been a Level 1.

Often, patients who are left with their illness unfolding and intricate changes unassessed can move from a Level 5 to a Level 1 quickly. The resiliency of a patient can be enhanced when the nursing characteristic of clinical inquiry is present at a high level.

REFERENCES

AACN. (2003). *Characteristics of Patients, Clinical Units and Systems of Concern to Nurse.* Available at: http://www.aacn.org/certcorp/certcorp.nsf/syn model. Accessed April 26, 2004.

Callahan, H. E. (2003). Families Dealing with Advanced Heart Failure: A Challenge and an Opportunity. *Critical Care Nursing Quarterly* 26(3): 230–243.

Curley, M. A. Q. (1998). Patient-Nurse Synergy: Optimizing Patients' Outcomes. *American Journal of Critical Care* 7(1): 64–72.

Doane, L. (2002). Overview of Tumor Lysis Syndrome. *Seminars in Oncology Nursing* 18(3): 2–5.

Felten, B. S. (2001). Resilience in Diverse Community-Dwelling Women Over Age 85. The University of Wisconsin–Milwaukee, doctoral dissertation.

Felten, B. S., and Hall, J. M. (2001). Conceptualizing Resilience in Women Older than 85: Overcoming Adversity from Illness or Loss. *Journal of Gerontological Nursing* 27(11): 46–53.

Gobel, B. H. (2002). Management of Tumor Lysis Syndrome: Prevention and Treatment. *Seminars in Oncology Nursing* 18(3): 12–16.

Greene, R. R. (2002). Holocaust Survivors: A Study in Resilience. *Journal of Gerontological Social Work* 37(1): 3–18.

Humphreys, J. (2003). Resilience in Sheltered Battered Women. *Issues in Mental Health Nursing* 24(2): 137–152.

Kaplow, R. (2002). Pathophysiology, Signs and Symptoms of Acute Tumor Lysis Syndrome. *Seminars in Oncology Nursing* 18(3): 6–11.

Lauer, C. S. (2002). The Relevance of Resilience. *Modern Healthcare* 32(33): 29.

Lothe, E. A., and Heggen, K. (2003). A Study of Resilience in Young Ethiopian Famine Survivors. *Journal of Transcultural Nursing* 14(4): 313–320.

Miller, D. B., and MacIntosh, R. (1999). Promoting Resilience in Urban African American Adolescents: Racial Socialization and Identity Theory as Promoting Factors. *Social Work Research* 23(3): 159–169.

Poblete, S. A. (2000). Relationship of Spirituality, Social Support, Reciprocity, and Conflict to Resilience in Individuals Diagnosed with HIV. Rutgers, The State University of New Jersey–Newark, doctoral dissertation.

Resiliency in Action, Inc. (2002). Available at: http://www.resiliency.com. Accessed February 3, 2003.

Talsma, A. N. (1995). An Evaluation of a Theoretical Model of Resilience and Select Predictors of Resilience in a Sample of Community-Based Elderly. The University of Michigan, doctoral dissertation.

Tusaie-Mumford, K. R. (2001). Psychosocial Resilience in Rural Adolescents: Optimism, Perceived Social Support and Gender Differences. The University of Pittsburgh, doctoral dissertation.

Wagnild, G. M., and Young, H. M. (1993). Development and Psychometric Evaluation of the Resilience Scale. *Journal of Nursing Measurement* 1(2): 165–178.

Werner, E. E., and Smith, R. S. (1992). *Overcoming the Odds: High Risk Children from Birth to Adulthood.* Ithaca, NY: Cornell University Press.

Woodgate, R. L. (1999). A Review of Literature on Resilience in the Adolescent with Cancer: Part II. *Journal of Pediatric Oncology Nursing* 16(2): 78–89.

CHAPTER 3

VULNERABILITY

Roberta Kaplow, PhD, RN, CCNS, CCRN

INTRODUCTION

The concept of vulnerability has been addressed in the literature from a number of perspectives. One outlook is the evaluation of "vulnerable populations." Some of these are identified based on socioeconomic status, ethnicity gender, and diagnosis (e.g., HIV/AIDS) (Flaskerud and Lee, 2001), age, and corresponding loss of physical functioning (Hennen and Knudten, 2001). Other sources of vulnerability are derived from prejudice, insensitivity to human rights, and failure to appreciate others' perspectives (Chinn, 2000). The term vulnerability has also been utilized in the social sciences literature addressing disaster, famine, and mental health (Delor and Hubert, 2000).

The process of caregiving has been identified as one of the factors that creates a situation of vulnerability. Research findings support that vulnerability is "composed of factors of anxiety, inferiority, insecurity, lack of intimacy, and disconfirmation" (Lidell et al., 1998, p. 72).

A number of situations can make a person vulnerable. These situations can occur in "anyone who is feeling threatened and uncertain" (Ebersole, 2002, p. 4). One such situation could be admission to an intensive care unit (ICU). McKinley and colleagues (2002) performed a qualitative study of seriously ill patients in an ICU. The data revealed sources of vulnerability in this patient sample that included extreme physical and emotional dependency, lack of information, and depersonalized care. The researchers concluded that feelings of vulnerability diminished when patients were kept informed of their status, were provided explanations about care they were to receive, when care was individualized based on their respective needs, and when families were present. These findings are consistent with other reported factors associated with vulnerability, including victimization, insecurity, and risk (Delor and Hubert, 2000).

A number of the factors related to patients' levels of vulnerability include their relationship with primary care practitioners (Shi et al., 2003); health variability

(Karpati et al., 2002); and transition in health care delivery with shorter length of hospital stay (Walker, 2001).

The literature also has focused on sequela of vulnerability. Outcomes such as quality of life (Sorensen and Pinquart, 2000; Spiers, 2000), adjustments to an operative procedure (Behel et al., 2002; van Servellan et al., 2002), and increased morbidity and mortality (Kurz, 2002) have all been linked to vulnerability.

DEFINITION

A number of industry definitions of vulnerability and vulnerable patients pervade the nursing literature. One such definition is "the susceptibility to particular harmful agents, conditions, or events at particular times and is considered something to be avoided or resisted" (Malone, 2000, p. 1). Another definition relevant to this chapter is "the inability to retain control of their life situations and/or to protect themselves against threats to their integrity (physical, emotional, wholeness, intactness)" (Irurita, 1999, p. 10).

The AACN Synergy Model definition of *vulnerability* is the susceptibility to actual or potential stressors that may adversely affect patient outcomes (Curley, 1998). A Level 1 patient is highly vulnerable, susceptible, unprotected, and fragile. A Level 3 patient is moderately vulnerable, somewhat susceptible, and somewhat protected. A Level 5 patient is minimally vulnerable, is safe, out of the woods, and not fragile (Kaplow, 2003; AACN, 2003).

CASE STUDY

CY is a 36-year-old male patient with no significant past medical history except for a recent shoulder injury. Social history revealed he was a one-pack-per-day tobacco smoker. He was admitted to the intensive care unit via the emergency department after an "attempted suicide" when he had ingested and overdosed on pain pills. Further exploration of his reason for overdosing revealed that he had a court date later that day for a credit card scam for which he admitted his guilt. He further admitted that he ingested the pills to avoid going to jail.

The paramedics intubated CY prior to transport to the hospital. In the emergency department, he was successfully treated for the overdose and was subsequently transferred to the intensive care unit for posttreatment monitoring and respiratory management.

CY remained intubated for 24 hours and had been stabilized and extubated. When he was ready for discharge from the hospital, the intensivist contacted the police per their request. As the police were literally walking into the unit to take CY into custody, it was noted that he had snuck out of the unit and escaped into a waiting car.

It was later learned that the police caught up with CY. He was transported to prison to await trial and continued to complain about shoulder pain. CY received medication to relieve the pain, but later was found in his prison cell unresponsive. He was transported back to the hospital and the ICU with an admitting diagnosis of aspiration pneumonia. CY hoarded the pain pills he was receiving and attempted another overdose. He remained intubated and on mechanical ventilation with antibiotic coverage for 10 days. During this admission, he was shackled to the bed with security at both doors to the ICU. Once again, he was stabilized and discharged in the custody of law enforcement officers.

APPLICATION OF THE CASE STUDY TO THE SYNERGY MODEL

In this scenario, during his first admission to the ICU, CY demonstrated moderate levels of resiliency. This is evidenced by his ability to compensate and respond to therapies. He was able to be extubated within 24 hours of his event. He initially demonstrated high levels of vulnerability but this diminished as he received therapies. CY was moderately stable and he was able to maintain a steady state for a limited period of time. He exhibited low levels of resource availability because he did not receive adequate psychological support. This is evidenced by a second suicide attempt. Patients with depressive episodes have a high vulnerability to reattempt suicide.

Given this lack of support, CY's second suicide attempt was predictable. He remained in a highly vulnerable state from a psychological perspective despite his moderate level of vulnerability from a physiologic perspective. Psychosocial approaches to care can significantly contribute to prevention of problems in the future.

During CY's second stay in the intensive care unit, the nurses caring for him demonstrated high levels of collaboration. They actively sought out contributions of other health care team members, including respiratory therapy and social work. They also involved law enforcement representatives, as required. Perhaps, collaboration with members of the psychosocial team would have been feasible if more time had been available.

Consistent with the AACN Synergy Model, Irurita (1999) suggests that patients having different levels of vulnerability to a health care situation and nursing interventions should be directed at promoting optimal patient outcomes. Admission to the ICU is often voluntary. However, if nurses are sensitive to the degree of vulnerability a patient brings to a health care situation, they play a pivotal role in identifying patients at risk for negative outcomes related to their vulnerability and can intervene as indicated.

REFERENCES

AACN. (2003). *Characteristics of Patients, Clinical Units and Systems of Concern to Nurse.* Available at: http://www.aacn.org/certcorp/certcorp.nsf/ synmodel. Accessed April 26, 2004.

Behel, J. M., Rybarczyk, B., Elliott, T., Nicholas, J. J., and Nyenhuis, D. (2002). The Role of Perceived Vulnerability in Adjustment to Lower Extremity Amputation: A Preliminary Investigation. *Rehabilitation Psychology* 47(1): 92–105.

Chinn, P. L. (2000). Not All Vulnerabilities Are Equal. *Advances in Nursing Science* 22(4): v.

Curley, M. A. Q. (1998). Patient-Nurse Synergy: Optimizing Patients' Outcomes. *American Journal of Critical Care* 7(1): 64–72.

Delor, F., and Hubert, M. (2000). Revisiting the Concept of 'Vulnerability.' *Social Science and Medicine* 50(1): 1557–1570.

Ebersole, P. (2002). Situational Vulnerability. *Geriatric Nursing* 23(1): 4–5.

Flaskerud, J. H., and Lee, P. (2001). Vulnerability to Health Problems in Female Informal Caregivers of Persons with HIV/AIDS and Age-Related Dementias. *Journal of Advanced Nursing* 33(1): 60–68.

Hennen, J. R., and Knudten, R. D. (2001). A Lifestyle Analysis of the Elderly: Perceptions of Risk, Fear, and Vulnerability. *Illness, Crisis, Loss* 9(2): 190–208.

Irurita, V. F. (1999). The Problem of Patient Vulnerability. *Collegian: Journal of the Royal College of Nursing, Australia* 6(1): 10–15.

Kaplow, R. (2003). AACN Synergy Model for Patient Care: A Framework to Optimize Outcomes. *Critical Care Nurse* 23(Suppl): 27–30.

Karpati, A., Galea, S., Awerbuch, T., and Levins, R. (2002). Variability, Vulnerability at the Ecological Level: Implications for Understanding the Social Determinants of Health. *American Journal of Public Health* 92(11): 1768–1772.

Kurz, J. M. (2002). Vulnerability of Well Spouses Involved in Lung Transplantation. *Journal of Family Nursing* 8(4): 353–370.

Lidell, R., Fridlund, B., and Segesten, K. (1998). Vulnerability Factors from a Pre- and Post-MI Perspective: A Qualitative Analysis. *Coronary Health Care* 2(2): 72–80.

Malone, R. E. (2000). Dimensions of Vulnerability in Emergency Nurses' Narratives. *Advances in Nursing Science* 23(1): 1–11.

McKinley, S., Nagy, S., Stein-Parbury, J., Bramwell, M., and Hudson, J. (2002). Vulnerability and Security in Seriously Ill Patients in Intensive Care. *Intensive and Critical Care* 18(1): 27–36.

Shi, L., Forrest, C. B., von Schrader, S., and Ng, J. (2003). Vulnerability and the Patient-Practitioner Relationship: The Roles of Gatekeeping and Primary Care Performance. *American Journal of Public Health* 93(1): 138–144.

Sorensen, S., and Pinquart, M. (2000). Vulnerability and Access to Resources as Predictors of Preparation for Future Care Needs in the Elderly. *Journal of Aging and Health* 12(3): 275–300.

Spiers, J. (2000). New Perspectives on Vulnerability Using Emie and Etic Approaches. *Journal of Advanced Nursing* 31(3): 715–721.

van Servellan, G., Chang, B., and Lombardi, E. (2002). Acculturation, Socioeconomic Vulnerability, and Quality of Life in Spanish-Speaking and Bilingual Latino HIV-Infected Men and Women. *Western Journal of Nursing Research* 24(3): 246–263.

Walker, A. (2001). Trajectory, Transition, and Vulnerability in Adult Medical-Surgical Patients: A Framework for Understanding In-Hospital Convalescence. *Contemporary Nurse* 11(2/3): 206–216.

CHAPTER 4

STABILITY

Roberta Kaplow, PhD, RN, CCNS, CCRN

INTRODUCTION

The limited literature addressing the concept of stability comes from few perspectives. One way it is addressed evaluates resources consumed by critically ill patients to maintain levels of stability. An example is the use of barbiturate coma in the management of increased intracranial pressure (Myles et al., 1996).

Patients' level of stability during hospitalization has also been used to predict morbidity and mortality rates and hospital recidivism. For example, in a study of patients hospitalized for pneumonia, those who had abnormal vital signs, confusion, or problems with eating or drinking in the 24 hours immediately prior to discharge had a higher mortality rate and had a higher likelihood of hospital readmission (Halm et al., 2002).

In a study of stability of urban family caregivers, stability was expressed in four themes. Caring expressions of stability were classified as:

1. emotional burden
2. evasion of conflicts
3. motivation from love and a sense of duty between caregivers, the care recipient, and their families
4. a filial, ethereal value

It was suggested that nurses integrate these expressions of stability into the rehabilitation process (Pierce, 2001).

DEFINITION

The AACN Synergy Model definition of *stability* is the ability to maintain a steady-state equilibrium (Curley, 1998). A Level 1 patient is minimally stable, is labile, unresponsive to therapies, and has a high risk for death. A Level 3 patient is moderately stable, is able to maintain a steady state for a limited period of time, and is somewhat responsive to therapies. A Level 5 patient is highly stable, is constant, is responsive to therapies, and is at a low risk for death (Kaplow, 2003; AACN, 2003).

CASE STUDY

SD is a 33-year-old female with a past medical history significant for Type I diabetes mellitus, depression, and anxiety. Her private physician treated her for a urinary tract infection 1 week prior to admission to the hospital. She presented to the emergency department with complaints of polyuria, polydipsia, and polyphagia, increasing weakness, mental cloudiness, and nausea. On physical exam, her skin was warm and dry, she was slightly tachypneic (RR = 30), had borderline hypotension (90/54), and Kussmaul respirations. The lab data were as follows:

Na	133
K	5.0
BUN	26
Creatinine	1.0
Glucose	420

The arterial blood gas revealed a metabolic acidosis. Urine was positive for ketones.

She was admitted to the intensive care unit with a diagnosis of diabetic ketoacidosis. SD was recently (2 days ago) discharged from the hospital after recovering from a similar event.

SD received 1 liter of 0.9% normal saline over 1 hour, a bolus of regular insulin of 10 units, followed by an insulin infusion starting at 0.1 unit/kg/hour, titrated hourly based on a blood glucose monitoring computer. She also received KCl 40 mEq in the first liter of IV fluids. Her maintenance IV was changed to $\frac{1}{2}$ NS with 5cc KPO_4 (22mEq K + 15mm Phosphorus)/liter at a rate of 300 ml/hour.

SD's blood sugar was normalized at a rate of 10 percent per hour to avoid complications of rapidly decreasing glucose. Her electrolytes and acid-base status normalized as well and SD was stabilized within 48 hours and was ready for discharge to the general medical unit.

Shortly after being admitted to the general medical unit, SD signed out of the hospital against medical advice. She returned to the hospital for the third time 3 days later, in a state of diabetic ketoacidosis.

APPLICATION OF THE CASE STUDY TO THE SYNERGY MODEL

Diabetic ketoacidosis is a complication of diabetes mellitus. It is caused by the build-up of ketones, which occurs when glucose is not available for body energy. When glucose is not available, body fat is broken down instead. The by-products of fat metabolism are ketones. When fat is metabolized, the blood becomes more acidic than body tissues. Blood glucose levels become elevated because the liver produces glucose to try to compensate for the problem. The cells cannot take up the glucose without insulin (which is lacking in diabetes mellitus) (Mehler, 1992).

In this scenario, upon admission, SD exhibited moderate levels of vulnerability and low levels of stability given her condition. She presented with classic signs of diabetic ketoacidosis. With aggressive therapy of intravenous hydration, insulin, and electrolyte supplementation, she was stabilized. She did not suffer any complications related to the blood glucose correction or electrolyte abnormalities (e.g., hypocalcemia secondary to phosphate binding). By virtue of her ability to stabilize, SD demonstrated moderate levels of resiliency as well. She was able to mount and maintain a response to therapies for a long enough time to be transferred from the ICU. SD exhibited high levels of predictability. She responded to therapies in the predicted way and followed a predictable clinical course. However, her stability level can be considered only moderate, because a few days later, she presented to the hospital with the same diagnosis. She was able to maintain a steady state for only a limited amount of time. If SD were able to sustain her blood sugar within normal limits, she would have exhibited a high level of stability, because she was responsive to therapies.

It is possible that if SD did not sign herself out against medical advice, she would have been able to receive some patient education to prevent future events. This might have led to a better outcome.

REFERENCES

AACN. (2003). *Characteristics of Patients, Clinical Units and Systems of Concern to Nurse.* Available at: http://www.accn.org/certcorp/certcorp.nsf/synmodel. Accessed April 26, 2004.

Curley, M. A. Q. (1998). Patient-Nurse Synergy: Optimizing Patients' Outcomes. *American Journal of Critical Care* 7(1): 64–72.

Halm, E. A., Fine, M. J., Kapoor, W. N., Singer, D. E., Marrie, T. J., and Siu, A. L. (2002). Instability on Hospital Discharge and the Risk of Adverse Outcomes in Patients with Pneumonia. *Archives of Internal Medicine* 162: 1278–1284.

Kaplow, R. (2003). AACN Synergy Model for Patient Care: A Framework to Optimize Outcomes. *Critical Care Nurse* 23(Suppl): 27–30.

Mehler, P. S. (1992). Diabetic Ketoacidosis. In P. E. Parsons and Wiener-Kronish, J. P. (eds.). *Critical Care Secrets.* Philadelphia: Hanley & Belfus, pp. 241–245.

Myles, G. L., Malkoff, M. D., Perry, A. G., Bucholz, R. D., and Gomez, C. R. (1996). Therapeutic Intervention Scoring System Used in the Care of Patients in Pentobarbital-Induced Coma to Determine Nurse-Patient Ratios. *American Journal of Critical Care* 5(1): 74–79.

Pierce, L. L. (2001). Caring and Expressions of Stability by Urban Family Caregivers of Persons with Stroke Within African American Family Systems. *Rehabilitation Nursing* 26(3): 100–107.

CHAPTER 5

COMPLEXITY

Roberta Kaplow, PhD, RN, CCNS, CCRN

INTRODUCTION

Patient complexity is often reported in the literature in a variety of ways. Information on patient complexity is important because changes in nursing interventions may be indicated based on a patient's clinical status. An example is the use of standards for pain management based on the complexity of the patient's pain (Lynch and Abrahm, 2002). Patients with graft-versus-host disease, a complication of allogenic bone marrow transplantation, are complex and require high levels of care consistent with the patient acuity (Bonavita et al., 2002). The same is true for patients with multiple organ dysfunction syndrome in the intensive care unit. These patients, depending on the number of organs involved and the degree of involvement, will have varying levels of complexity.

A study of medically complex premature children was conducted to evaluate feeding difficulties in this group. It was found that medically premature children, especially those who needed respiratory support, experienced feeding difficulties. It was suggested that these children would benefit from ongoing oral-motor feeding interventions (Burklow et al., 2002).

Complexity from a psychosocial perspective is also examined. One of the more challenging circumstances is a family discussion surrounding withdrawal and withholding of therapies in the intensive care unit (ICU). Communication approaches and support that is provided to the family during these difficult times should reflect the complexity of the situation (Curtis et al., 2002).

Complexity is also addressed in the literature in terms of intricacy of therapies or treatment regimens. The advent of newer modes of mechanical ventilation for the treatment of acute respiratory distress syndrome (McKinley et al., 2001) and use of emerging combination therapies for HIV/AIDS (Frame, 2003) based on enhanced knowledge bases in these respective areas are examples of complexity of therapies and how they impact patient care.

The complexity of the role of the parent as caregiver for a child with cancer is delved into as well. The challenges of parents involve many processes including protection of their identity and that of their child (Young et al., 2002), in addition to the physical and emotional support that is required during therapy.

Patients' actual complexity level is compared to nurses' perception of those same patients' complexity is explored in the literature. Use of these data can be used for resource allocation based on patient need (Donohue, 1993).

DEFINITION

Complexity is defined as the intricate entanglement of two or more systems (e.g., body, family, therapies) (Curley, 1998). Based on the tenets of the AACN Synergy Model, a Level 1 patient is highly complex, and intricate, and has complex patient/family dynamics or a vague, atypical presentation. A Level 3 patient has moderate patient/family dynamics. A Level 5 patient is simple, uncomplicated, has a clear-cut presentation, and has routine family dynamics (Kaplow, 2003; AACN, 2003).

CASE STUDY

CN is a 15-year-old patient admitted to the intensive care unit status post (s/p) allogeneic bone marrow transplant for aplastic anemia 5 days ago. She was admitted with a diagnosis of nadir sepsis. She was pancytopenic due to her pretransplant regimen. CN's parents are divorced and she is the second oldest of four children living with her father. Her mother left the father and the children several years ago.

CN's clinical course was complicated by bacterial pneumonia requiring prolonged mechanical ventilation and antibiotic therapy, hemodynamic instability requiring vigorous fluid resuscitation and vasopressor therapy, and renal insufficiency due to hypoperfusion. Due to her prolonged need for mechanical ventilation, CN required a tracheotomy.

CN's family dynamics presented a challenge for the multidisciplinary team of the intensive care unit. CN's father was argumentative, manipulative, unrelenting, and passive-aggressive. He was extremely controlling, wanting a say in every medical decision and wanting to regulate his daughter's medical care. Members of the multidisciplinary team, especially nurses and physicians, experienced great difficulty doing their work because the father placed multiple barriers for this to take place. He verbalized that he felt that rules applied to everyone but him.

The emotional turmoil the family dynamics created on a daily basis required frequent reassignment of nursing staff caring for CN. The concepts inherent in primary nursing and the AACN Synergy Model had to take a back seat in order to prevent an entire staff from resigning after feeling abused by the father.

CN was successfully treated for her bout of sepsis, respiratory failure, and renal insufficiency. She was subsequently discharged back to the pediatric unit and, several weeks later, was discharged from the hospital.

Four months later, CN was readmitted to the hospital with shortness of breath, dyspnea on exertion, weight loss, and decline in performance status. The skin on her face and upper extremities had a leathery appearance to it. She was intubated and placed on mechanical ventilation. According to her father who provided the most recent history, he had stopped giving CN the cyclosporine therapy, feeling "CN did not need it anymore." Mr. N admitted that his stopping the medication was not a financial issue because the insurance company was covering the therapy. Once again, he felt "the doctors don't know what they are talking about; they overexaggerate everything and that CN should not have to be on medicine any longer. The transplant was a success. That was all that my daughter needed."

CN was subsequently diagnosed with graft-versus-host disease (GVHD) in her lungs. GVHD is a potential complication of allogeneic bone marrow transplantation. Another course of prolonged mechanical ventilation ensued, necessitating CN to undergo a tracheostomy procedure once again. After 1 month in the ICU, it became apparent that CN would require long-term ventilatory support. She was otherwise stable. After several meetings with the multidisciplinary team and the father, it was decided to initiate procedures to prepare CN for discharge home. These plans included acclimating CN gradually to a home ventilator; extensive family teaching about suctioning, tracheostomy care, and other aspects of airway management; and coordinating the utilities company in CN's neighborhood so there would not be a disruption of electricity in CN's home in the event of a power shortage.

Mr. N continued to be an obstacle with all attempts at preparation for discharge. He refused to learn how to suction, perform trach care, or any aspect of CN's care. One of CN's sisters was amenable to learning. She, however, was in high school and could not assume full-time responsibility for CN's care. The other sisters refused to participate in caring for CN.

Ultimately, despite Mr. N's finding fault with every suggestion and alternative, arrangements were made for home health aides to care for CN. She was discharged home several weeks later.

APPLICATION OF THE CASE STUDY TO THE SYNERGY MODEL

GVHD is a possible complication of any allogeneic transplant (from a donor) and occurs when the donor's stem cells are establishing in the recipient's body. T-cells, one of the most powerful cells of the immune system, may begin to attack the recipient's body, acting directly on foreign materials in the body to kill them. GVHD is thought to occur when there is enough of a difference between the donor and recipient that the T-cells from the donor determine that the recipient's body is foreign (Rosenzweig, 1998).

CN's case was complex from a number of perspectives. She was diagnosed with a life-threatening illness, overcoming many obstacles from a physiologic perspective in preparation for her bone marrow transplant. Despite statistics and numerous posttransplant complications, she was successfully engrafted and was discharged home. The complexity of her situation was augmented by her family dynamics. Her mother was estranged for several years prior to her diagnosis and her father presented many barriers for the staff to care for her. Though admittingly lacking any medical background or knowledge, Mr. N discontinued her immunosuppressive therapy, which resulted in GVHD. Further compounding the complexity of the situation was the division of CN's immediate family in terms of their willingness to care for her at home. She will likely spend the remainder of her life ventilator-dependent. This has implications for how she will continue her education, have a social life, as well as all other aspects of a "normal" life.

All members of the health care team exhibited high levels of clinical judgment during CN's course in the intensive care unit. She survived a critical event, was successfully treated for her pneumonia, and was stabilized to the point of being able to be discharged home on mechanical ventilation. The nursing staff exhibited high levels of clinical inquiry by implementing open visitation for the family and providing them with frequent updates on CN's condition. The nursing staff also demonstrated high levels as facilitators of learning by attempting to teach the patient and cooperative family members tracheostomy care and suctioning techniques.

REFERENCES

AACN. (2003). *Characteristics of Patients, Clinical Units and Systems of Concern to Nurse.* Available at: http://www.aacn.org/certcorp/certcorp.nsf/ syn model. Accessed April 26, 2004.

Bonavita, K. K., Marsullo, M., and Rasero, L. (2002). Acute GVHD: A Retrospective Analysis of 55 Bone Marrow Transplant Patients. *Assistenza Infermieristica e Ricerca: Air* 21(4): 193–197.

Burklow, K. A., McGrath, A. M., Valerius, K. S., and Rudolph, C. (2002). Relationship Between Feeding Difficulties, Medical Complexity, and Gestational Age. *Nutrition in Clinical Practice* 17(6): 373–378.

Curley, M. A. Q. (1998). Patient-Nurse Synergy: Optimizing Patients' Outcomes. *American Journal of Critical Care* 7(1): 64–72.

Curtis, J. R., Engelberg, R. A., Wenrich, M. D., Nielsen, E. L., Shannon, S. E., Treece, P. D., Tonelli, M. R., Patrick, D. L., Robins, L. S., McGrath, B. B., and Rubenfeld, G. D. (2002). Studying Communication About End-of-Life During the ICU Family Conference: Development of a Framework. *Journal of Critical Care* 17(3): 147–160.

Donohue, R. K. (1993). Patient Care Classification Systems: A Study in Home Care. *Journal of Home Health Care Practice* 5(2): 20–37.

Frame, P. T. (2003). HIV Disease in Primary Care. *Primary Care: Clinics of Office Practice* 30(1): 205–237.

Kaplow, R. (2003). AACN Synergy Model for Patient Care: A Framework to Otimize Outcomes. *Critical Care Nurse* 23(Suppl): 27–30.

Lynch, M., and Abrahm, J. (2002). Ensuring a Good Death: Pain and Palliative Care in a Cancer Center. *Cancer Practice* 10 Suppl(1): S33–38.

McKinley, B. A., Moore, F. A., Sailors, R. M., Cocanour, C. S., Marquez, A., Wright, R. K., Tonnesen, A. S., Wallace, C. J., Morris, A. H., and East, T. D. (2001). Computerized Decision Support for Mechanical Ventilation of Trauma Induced ARDS: Results of a Randomized Clinical Trial. *Journal of Trauma-Injury Infection and Critical Care* 50(3): 415–425.

Rosenzweig, M. Q. (1998). Graft vs. Host Disease. In C. C. Chernecky and B. J. Berger (eds.). *Advanced and Critical Care Oncology Nursing*. Philadelphia: WB Saunders Co., pp. 172–188.

Young, B., Dixon-Woods, M., and Heney, D. (2002). Identity and Role in Parenting a Child with Cancer. *Rehabilitation* 5(4): 209–214.

CHAPTER 6

RESOURCE AVAILABILITY

Roberta Kaplow, PhD, RN, CCNS, CCRN

INTRODUCTION

The family is an essential factor in the course, outcomes, treatment, and care of the health and illness of its individual members (D'Cruz, 2003). It is also essential for the prevention of problem behaviors and promotion of psychosocial behaviors (Kerr et al., 2003). Nurses have an understanding of the resource availability of patients from vulnerable populations (e.g., homeless) for the purpose of diagnosing and treating health problems (Strehlow and Amos-Jones, 1999).

One of the frequently evaluated resources that a patient brings to a clinical picture is human resources—family and significant others. There are inconsistent findings in the literature regarding a reduction in resource use and increased use of comfort measures in patients as they are dying (Kaplow, 1998; Tschann et al., 2003). In one study, patients who had a family member present at the time of death also had a shorter time between the writing of a do-not-resuscitate order and the actual time of death. One of the factors that impacted on a patient at the end of life with decision making was the patient's social network (Sahlberg-Blom et al., 2000).

Upon evaluation of a family-directed program designed to prevent adolescent tobacco use, it was found that the program was effective in reducing the onset of smoking in the population studied (Bauman et al., 2001). Conversely, in a study of patients with diabetes, social support was not strongly related to diabetes self-management (Gleeson-Kreig et al., 2002).

In a study of patients s/p bone marrow transplantation, one of the factors that significantly impacted patient survival was social support stability (Rodrigue et al., 1999). In another study, muscle strength and mobility improved in patients with hemiplegia from stroke when family members participated in care (Maeshima et al., 2003). In a different study of stroke patients, it was revealed that lay caregivers and patients need to receive information and education on treatment and rehabilitation (Portillo-Vega et al., 2002). It has also been suggested that permitting parental visitation in the operating room for induction of anesthesia may decrease stress associated with separation occurring in pediatric patients (Nash and Murphy, 1997).

DEFINITION

Based on the AACN Synergy Model, *resource availability* is defined as the extent of resources (personal, financial, social, psychological, technical, etc.) the patient, family, and community bring to the current situation (AACN, 2003; Curley, 1998; Mullen, 2002). A Level 1 patient has few resources; necessary knowledge and skill are not available. The patient has minimal personal/psychological supportive resources, and few social systems available. A Level 3 patient is considered to have moderate resources. This patient has limited knowledge and skill available, limited financial resources available, limited personal and psychological supportive resources, and limited social systems. A Level 5 patient has many resources: Extensive knowledge and skills are available and accessible and financial resources are readily available, as well as strong personal and psychological supportive resources and strong social systems and resources.

A patient's clinical situation can be impacted based on availability of resources. Limited availability of resources can constrain a patient's recovery from a critical illness or event.

CASE STUDY

BG is a 90-year-old patient with a history of polycythemia vera, back pain, and numbness in both lower extremities due to spinal stenosis, osteoarthritis, benign prostate hypertrophy (BPH), and macular degeneration. BG lost his wife, the matriarch of the family, 6 years ago. Since then, he has lived in a cluttered, infested apartment. Most recently, he agreed to board two drug users in his apartment in the hope that they would be able to assist him with some of his activities of daily living. He needed the most help with shopping, moving his car (city parking has alternate side of the street parking regulations), and being driven to the cemetery to visit his wife (which he insisted on doing daily since his wife's death).

Not surprisingly, BG's roommates began stealing from him. Several of his wife's personal items were pawned for the purchase of illegal drugs. Food in the house was rancid and BG was rarely taken to the cemetery to visit his wife's gravesite. He was "forced" to drive himself to the site, driving between lanes because of his impaired vision. BG had difficulty walking and maintaining his balance without the use of a cane because of the persistent numbness in his legs and feet.

BG refused help from his family. He has two married daughters and several adult grandchildren all who, despite living out of town, frequently offered him a home with them or to visit and help him. He refused all help from his family because he "didn't want to burden them." He frequently told them not to come visit, that "it would be too much for me if you come up."

BG presented to his physician with an upper respiratory infection, for which oral antibiotics were prescribed. Two days into therapy, BG developed difficulty swallowing the pills and consequently stopped taking the antibiotics as well as the medication he was taking for BPH. Two days later, he developed abdominal pain. He was found to have a distended bladder and was admitted to the hospital. He was diagnosed with hydronephrosis, hyperkalemia, and renal insufficiency.

BG's hyperkalemia was successfully treated with sodium polystyrene sulfonate (Kayexalate®). His clinical status appeared to be stable and he was discharged to a rehabilitation facility. Three days postdischarge, he was readmitted to the hospital in acute renal failure secondary to dehydration. BG had stopped eating and drinking because of severe back pain. Upon admission, his WBC was 20,000; he was febrile, hyperkalemic, and oliguric. He was admitted to the ICU for management. A hemodialysis catheter was inserted and treatments were initiated. Dialysis treatments were complicated by episodes of hemodynamic instability that responded to fluid resuscitation.

Late one afternoon, BG went into cardiac arrest and resuscitative measures were instituted. During the code, BG's two daughters arrived to visit. Based on their expressed wishes, resuscitative efforts were terminated.

APPLICATION OF THE CASE STUDY TO THE SYNERGY MODEL

Since his wife's death, BG had low levels of resource availability. This was somewhat self-imposed because he had many caring family members who repeatedly offered to assist him. When he became ill, BG exhibited high levels of complexity, vulnerability, and instability. He initially demonstrated some degree of resiliency when he recovered from his first episode of hyperkalemia.

It was since his wife's death that BG's level of health began to decline. He had limited availability of resources that he chose to use. This partially contributed to his impaired recovery from critical illness. Ironically, he was able to die with his family at his bedside.

The nurses caring for BG in this situation exhibited high levels of clinical judgment and caring practices. They also demonstrated high levels of clinical inquiry by allowing the family to remain with BG during the resuscitative efforts until they decided to have them terminated. This is consistent with the American Heart Association guidelines (www.americanheart.org) that recommend family members be offered the opportunity to stay with the patient during cardiopulmonary resuscitation. It is suggested in the literature that nurses focus on the patient's family and significant others in interventions for health, illness, and prevention (D'Cruz, 2003).

REFERENCES

AACN. (2003). *Characteristics of Patients, Clinical Units and Systems of Concern to Nurse.* Available at: http://www.aacn.org/certcorp/certcorp.nsf/syn model. Accessed April 26, 2004.

Bauman, K. E., Foushee, V. A., Ennett, S. T., Pemberton, M., Hicks, K. A., King, T. S., and Koch, G. G. (2001). The Influence of a Family Program on Adolescent Tobacco and Alcohol Use. *American Journal of Public Health* 91(4): 604–610.

Curley, M. A. Q. (1998). Patient-Nurse Synergy: Optimizing Patients' Outcomes. *American Journal of Critical Care* 7(1): 64–72.

D'Cruz, P. (2003). Family Focused Interventions in Health and Illness. *Journal of Health Management* 5(1): 37–56.

Gleeson-Kreig, J., Bernal, H., and Woolley, S. (2002). The Role of Social Support in the Self-Management of Diabetes Mellitus Among a Hispanic Population. *Public Health Nursing* 19(3): 215–222.

Kaplow, R. (1998). An Exploration of the Relationship Between Nursing Resource Use and Comfort in Cancer Patients in the ICU With and Without a DNR Order. New York University, doctoral dissertation.

Kerr, M. H., Beck, K., Shattuck, T. D., Kattar, C., and Uriburu, D. (2003). Family Involvement, Problem and Prosocial Behavior Outcomes of Latino Youth. *American Journal of Health Behavior* 27 Suppl(1): S55–65.

Maeshima, S., Ueyoshi, A., Osawa, A., Ishida, K., Kunimoto, K., Shimamoto, Y., Matsumoto, T., and Yoshida, M. (2003). Mobility and Muscle Strength Contralateral to Hemiplegia from Stroke: Benefit from Self-Training with Family Support. *American Journal of Physical Medicine and Rehabilitation* 82(6): 456–462.

Mullen, J. E. (2002). The Synergy Model as a Framework for Nursing Rounds. *Critical Care Nurse* 22(6): 66–68.

Nash, P. A. L., and Murphy, J. M. (1997). An Approach to Pediatric Perioperative Care: Parent-Present Induction. *Nursing Clinics of North America* 32(1): 183–199.

Portillo-Vega, M. C., Wilson-Bartnett, J., and Saracibar-Razquin, M. I. (2002). Study of Patients' and Families' Perception of Lay Caregiver Participation in the Care of Stroke Patients: Methodology and Preliminary Results. *Enfermeria Clinica* 12(3): 94–103.

Rodrigue, J. R., Pearman, T. P., and Moreb, J. (1999). Morbidity and Mortality Following Bone Marrow Transplantation: Predictive Utility of Pre-BMT Affective Functioning, Compliance, and Social Support Stability. *International Journal of Behavioral Medicine* 6(3): 241–254.

Sahlberg-Blom, E., Ternestedt, B., and Johansson, J. (2000). Patient Participation in Decision Making at the End of Life as Seen by a Close Relative. *Nursing Ethics: An International Journal for Health Care Professionals* 7(4): 296–313.

Strehlow, A. J., and Amos-Jones, T. (1999). The Homeless as a Vulnerable Population. *Nursing Clinics of North America* 34(2): 261–274.

Tschann, J. M., Kaufman, S. R., and Micco, G. P. (2003). Family Involvement in End-of-Life Hospital Care. *Journal of the American Geriatrics Society* 51(6): 835–840.

C H A P T E R 7

PARTICIPATION IN CARE

Roberta Kaplow, PhD, RN, CCNS, CCRN

INTRODUCTION

Decisions related to health care are complex (Kravitz and Melnikov, 2001), and patient participation is considered valuable and beneficial in the nursing literature. This expression has been used interchangeably with patient involvement, partnership, and collaboration. Given that there needs to be collaboration between the patient and nurse, this presumes that patients need to be central to decisions that affect their health and well-being (Jewell, 1994).

A growing trend exists of patients participating in their care. Patients are assuming more accountability for prevention and treatment of health problems, and this participation augments or replaces care by professionals (Cahill, 1998).

The value and importance of family participation in care is well documented (Henderson and Shum, 2003; Kjelin et al., 2002; Portillo-Vega et al., 2002). Given this importance, participation in care has become increasingly accepted in nursing practice (Cahill, 1998).

There is a plethora of data supporting parental participation in the care of children; care that has been found to be quite valuable (Kjelin et al., 2002). Investigators of one qualitative study reported that parents wish to participate in care of their children and prefer to select the degree of their participation (Neill, 1996). There is reported variability in how patients conceptualized participation in care. Some believed it meant contributing to decisions or expressing views of treatment options (Sainio et al., 2001); there is also reported inconsistency of expectations of participation in care between parents and nurses. Parents in one study expected to have a higher level of participation (Blower and Morgan, 2000), while in another study, parents preferred to participate in activities of daily living and have the professionals be responsible for the child's clinical care (Neill, 1996).

Patient participation in care was enhanced by a number of factors: good health, access to information, assertiveness, high-quality interactions with nurses and physicians, and encouragement by these health care providers to participate (Sainio et al., 2001). In another study, nurses who were parents, married, or cared for patients with burns, on a craniofacial unit, or in a general surgery unit had a more accepting attitude of parental participation in care than staff on other units or who did not have these demographic characteristics (Johnson and Lindschau, 1996).

Factors reported to have impeded patients' participation in care include poor health, ignorance, anxiety, age, time pressures by staff, lack of time, high staff turnover, and poor interactive relationships (Melnyk and Feinstein, 2001; Sainio et al., 2001). Factors that impeded parental participation in care included the relationships between the parents and the professionals, short hospital admissions, and single hospital admissions (Neill, 1996).

Outcomes of parental participation in care have also been evaluate. In one study, parents who wished to participate in care believed their child was experiencing less pain as compared to parents who did not want as much participation (Kristensoon-Hallstrom, 1999).

Outcomes of participation in care reported in the literature include decreased anxiety (Littlefield et al., 1990); enhanced decision making, human dignity, and quality of life (Cahill, 1998); and increased patient satisfaction and compliance (Jewell, 1994).

DEFINITION

The Synergy Model definition of *participation in care* is the extent to which the patient and family engage in care (Curley, 1998). A Level 1 patient and family have no participation. They have no capacity or desire for decision making. A Level 3 patient and family have moderate levels of participation. They have limited capacity and seek advice from others in decision making. Often, advice may be sought from friends or neighbors. These individuals may quote something they have seen on television or read on the Internet and may not have accurate data. A Level 5 patient and family fully participates in decision making. The patient and family have capacity and can make decisions for themselves (Kaplow, 2003). At Level 5, the patient and family actively seek information, are open to instruction, and desire an active role in the delivery of care to a family member.

CASE STUDY

SC is a 62-year-old male patient with a history of mild hypertension, hypercholesterolemia, and mitral regurgitation status post myocardial infarction. He presented to the emergency department with shortness of breath, dyspnea on exertion, episodes of dizziness, edema in both feet and ankles, and ease of fatigue. He reported mild to moderate limitations with his activities of daily living. Chest X-rays revealed acute pulmonary edema and right lower lobe pneumonia. Echocardiogram revealed an approximate ejection fraction of 15 percent.

SC was admitted to the coronary care unit for management of heart failure and further observation. He was treated with vigorous diuresis with furosemide (Lasix®) and inotropic support with dobutamine hydrochloride (Dobutrex®). Within 2 hours of admission, SC developed paroxysmal supraventricular tachycardia that was refractory to medications. He was sedated and successfully cardioverted into his baseline (admission) sinus tachycardia (rate of 108) with no further episodes of the tachyarrhythmia.

Upon assessment, the nurse caring for SC learned that he had not been adhering to his dietary sodium restriction. This and his other symptoms were associated with a 5-pound weight gain in the past week. The weight gain seemed to puzzle SC because he complained that his wife's cooking is "bland and boring," that it "had no taste anymore." He recalled being taught about some foods to avoid on a low-sodium diet. While taking a diet history of the previous week, in collaboration with his wife, it was determined that SC was not adherent with adding salt to foods even though Mrs. C was careful not to cook any food with additional salt. Salted snacks were forbidden in the house. Mrs. C stated that she eliminated those from her diet in support of her husband. The nurse collaborated with the unit-based nutritionist regarding SC.

The nurse caring for SC requested that the nutritionist meet with SC and his wife. The nutritionist met with them to determine their knowledge about foods to avoid in a sodium-restricted diet. The nutritionist also provided ideas for seasonings and marinades to be used in place of salt as well as instruction on how to read labels of prepared foods in the market. The nurses referred SC to available reading materials and to the American Heart Association Web site (www.americanheart.org) for further information. They also emphasized the importance of following a low-sodium diet appropriately. SC was stabilized and was transferred from the coronary care unit 2 days following admission. Once stabilized, SC continued on diuretics and was started on traditional medications to treat congestive heart failure, including an ACE-inhibitor enalapril (Vasotec®), potassium chloride (KCl), digoxin (Lanoxin®), and a beta-blocker, Carvedilol (Coreg®). His ECG remained unchanged and his cardiac enzymes remained normal. He was discharged home the following day. When seen again on a routine physician visit, SC was stable and asymptomatic. Mrs. C maintained her husband on a low-sodium diet by placing herself on one as well.

APPLICATION OF THE CASE STUDY TO THE SYNERGY MODEL

Heart failure occurred and the heart did not pump adequately to meet its demands because the muscle was damaged in SC's previous myocardial infarction (Lamborn et al., 2001). SC developed a tachyarrhythmia; this is common in heart failure because the heart attempts to compensate for abnormal blood flow by beating faster. This compensatory mechanism is only temporary and the heart cannot continue to meet the demands of the body. As a result, the cells, organs, muscles, and tissues in the body do not receive adequate amounts of oxygen. The decrease in oxygen to the kidneys results in sodium and water retention. This is what caused the weight gain and edematous feet and ankles seen in SC. In addition, SC's underlying cardiac condition (mitral valve regurgitation) coupled with the heart's inability to pump adequately caused fluid to back up from the left side of the heart to the lungs, resulting in the shortness of breath, dyspnea on exertion, and SC being easily fatigued. Blood can also back up in the abdomen, causing loss of appetite. A decrease in oxygen to the muscles results in feelings of tiredness.

In order to ensure optimal outcomes, patients must understand that they will need to continue to follow a sodium-restricted diet and continue to take their medications throughout their lifetime even if symptoms improve. Although there is no cure for chronic heart failure (except for transplant), participation in care by adhering to diet and medication regimen will ameliorate symptoms and help prevent complications and life-threatening events.

In this situation, Mr. C was admitted to the coronary care unit with low to moderate levels of stability and vulnerability. Given the frequency of patients admitted to the coronary care unit, SC was relatively high in terms of predictability. He responded well to therapies. He had relatively high levels of resource availability because Mrs. C was supportive of her husband and his treatment. SC also had a high level of participation in care. He provided all needed information and was honest and forthcoming about his lack of adherence to his sodium restriction. Mrs. C exhibited high levels of participation in his care as well by creating a home environment that was therapeutic in terms of dietary restrictions, changing her own diet to help support her husband. She listened to all of the advice provided by the nutritionist and successfully implemented them upon SC's discharge from the hospital. The interventions were successful, as evidenced by SC's health status at his next physician visit.

SC's stability is consistent with findings reported in the nursing literature. SC was able to remain out of the hospital due to his participation in care by following his sodium-restricted diet. This can be attributed to the education he and his wife received, his available social support, and openness to learning. Presence of these factors has contributed to prevention of hospitalization (Hardin and Hussey, 2003).

This positive outcome enforces the need for nurses to provide lay caregivers information on prevention and management of health conditions. When the patient is a child, clarification and negotiation of roles between the parent and the nurse is suggested so that everyone's expectations can be met (Blower and Morgan, 2000). One of the questions addressed in the literature is how nurses should intervene if family members are not willing or able to participate in care (Lee and Craft-Rosenberg, 2002). Suggestions for this dilemma need to be addressed.

Patients should be invited to be active collaborators rather than passive recipients of care. Nurses should look for ways to promote patient participation in care. Strategies should include promoting an environment conducive to patient questioning and commitment to providing answers to these questions in a manner that patients can understand (Jewell, 1994).

REFERENCES

Blower, K., and Morgan, E. (2000). Great Expectations? Parental Participation in Care. *Journal of Child Health Care* 4(2): 60–65.

Cahill, J. (1998). Patient Participation—A Review of Literature. *Journal of Clinical Nursing* 7(2): 119–128.

Curley, M. A. Q. (1998). Patient-Nurse Synergy: Optimizing Patients' Outcomes. *American Journal of Critical Care* 7(1): 64–72.

Hardin, S., and Hussey, L. (2003). AACN Synergy Model for Patient Care. Case Study of a CHF Patient. *Critical Care Nurse* 23(1): 73–76.

Henderson, A., and Shum, D. (2003). Decision-Making Preferences Toward Surgical Intervention in a Hong Kong Chinese Population. *International Nursing Review* 50(2): 95–100.

Jewell, S. E. (1994). Patient Participation: What Does It Mean to Nurses? *Journal of Advanced Nursing* 19: 433–438.

Johnson, A., and Lindschau, A. (1996). Staff Attitudes Toward Parent Participation in Care of Children Who Are Hospitalized. *Pediatric Nursing* 22(2): 99–102.

Kaplow, R. (2003). AACN Synergy Model for Patient Care: A Framework to Optimize Outcomes. *Critical Care Nurse* 23(1): 27–30.

Kjelin, A., Malmborg, M., and Hallstrom, I. (2002). Increased Parental Participation in Care of Boys Undergoing Surgery for Hypospadias Repair—Parents' Views. *Vard iI Norden. Nursing Science and Research in the Nordic Countries* 22(2): 38–42.

Kravitz, R. L., and Melnikov, J. (2001). Engaging Patients in Medical Decision Making. *British Medical Journal* 323(7313): 584–585.

Kristensson-Hallstrom, I. (1999). Strategies for Feeling Secure Influence Parents' Participation in Care. *Journal of Clinical Nursing* 8(5): 586–592.

Lamborn, M. L., Mosely, M. J., and Sole, M. L. (2001). Cardiac Alterations. In Sole, M. L., Lamborn, M. L., Hartshorn, J. C. (eds.). *Introduction to Critical Care Nursing,* 3rd ed. Philadelphia: WB Saunders Co., pp 239–282.

Lee, A., and Craft-Rosenberg, M. (2002). Ineffective Family Participation in Professional Care: A Concept Analysis of a Proposed Nursing Diagnosis. *Nursing Diagnosis* 13(1): 5–14.

Littlefield, V. M., Chang, A., and Adams, B. N. (1990). Participation in Alternative Care: Relationship to Anxiety, Depression, and Hostility. *Research in Nursing and Health* 13(1): 17–25.

Melnyk, B. M., and Feinstein, N. F. (2001). Mediating Functions of Maternal Anxiety and Participation in Care on Young Children's Posthospital Adjustment. *Research in Nursing and Health* 24(1): 18–26.

Neill, S. J. (1996). Parent Participation 1: Literature Review and Methodology. *British Journal of Nursing* 5(1): 34–40.

Portillo-Vega, M. C., Wilson-Bartnett, J., and Saracibar Razquin, M. I. (2002). Study of Patients' and Families' Perception of Lay Caregiver Participation in Care of Stroke Patients: Methodology and Preliminary Results. *Enfermeria Clinica* 12(3): 94–103.

Sainio, C., Lauri, S., and Eriksson, E. (2001). Cancer Patients' Views and Experiences of Participation in Care and Decision Making. *Nursing Ethics: An International Journal for Healthcare Professionals* 8(2): 97–113.

CHAPTER 8

PARTICIPATION IN DECISION MAKING

Roberta Kaplow, PhD, RN, CCNS, CCRN

INTRODUCTION

"The traditional concept of the doctor-patient relationship places the patient in a passive, dependent role with nothing to do but seek competent help and cooperate with the physician in order to get well" (Brody, 1980, p. 718). Until recently, it was an expectation that patients would be passive recipients of care (Biley, 1992). Now, participation in decision making is considered the foundation of ethical medical practice (Avis, 1994; Gattelari et al., 2002). However, patient participation in decision making has caused discussions among health care professionals (Sainio and Lauri, 2003). These include discussions related to the extent patients should participate in care and how to determine if patients are competent to make informed decisions about their care.

Patients in western cultures have been encouraged to participate in decision making related to health care issues for a number of reasons. These include economic, social, ethical, and legal concerns (Henderson and Shum, 2003). The literature on decision making reveals that patients prefer to be knowledgeable about treatment options and want to participate in decision making when treatment choices exist (Guadagnoli and Ward, 1998). In one study, women undergoing breast cancer treatment who participated in the decision making regarding treatment reported a higher level of posttreatment satisfaction (Sheehan, 1994). Conversely, patients reported a lower level of anxiety when not asked to participate in decision making during a visit with a urologist (Margalith and Shapiro, 1997). However, one reported outcome associated with increased patient participation in decision making was increased anxiety (Gattelari et al., 2002).

The degree to which patients wished to participate in decision making can range from the physician having full control to the individual having complete control. However, patients do not always wish to participate in decision making (Biley, 1992; Kravitz and Melnikov, 2001). In one study, patients preferred to have greater participation in decision making if the medical condition was not severe. Younger patients preferred to have greater collaboration with the physician than older patients (Henderson and Shum, 2003). In another study, when patients had more information about their condition, they wanted to participate more in the decision making (Barry and Henderson, 1996).

Inclination for active participation in decision making varies with cultural background and the clinical situation; at the very least, however, patients want to be informed (Kravitz and Melnikov, 2001). In one study, elderly patients representing varying ethnic backgrounds who were facing terminal illness were asked about their preference for information and involvement in decision making. African Americans and European Americans were more likely than Korean Americans and Mexican Americans to support patient autonomy for decision making. The latter two groups advocated for their families to hear about treatment options and for them to participate in medical decision making (Blackwell et al., 1995).

Issues related to patient participation in decision making, such as when the patient is a child, has sparked some controversy. Children are not consistently permitted to participate in decision making. Furthermore, it has been demonstrated that parents do not always back their child in complex circumstances. Health care providers do not consistently present alternatives to care or solicit a child's opinion about their care, but rather provide an explanation of what will transpire (Runeson et al., 2002). Health care providers do not agree as to what constitutes "old enough" for a child to participate in decision making (Shemmings, 2000).

Reported factors that had a positive impact on patient participation in decision making included good health, access to information, assertiveness, good interaction, relationships with nurses and physicians, and encouragement by these health care providers to participate (Sainio, Eriksson, and Lauri, 2001); patient participation in care (Cahill, 1998); patient's physical condition, marital status, and age (younger) (Thompson et al., 1993); time since diagnosis with cancer; information obtained by staff and relationships with staff (Sainio and Lauri, 2003); patient's activity, presence of a nurse/physician, treatment of patients as equals, and nurses and physicians having enough time for patients (Sainio, Eriksson, and Lauri, 2003). Patients were also more likely to participate in decision making when the nurse and physician promoted patient acquisition of information (Davidson, 1997), when patients had higher education, and when decisions did not require medical expertise (Thompson et al., 1993).

In one study, factors that impaired patients' participation in decision making included poor health, ignorance, anxiety, age, time pressures of staff, high staff turnover, and poor interactive relationships. Patients in this study were divided into three groups: (1) active participants, (2) those giving active consent, and (3) those giving passive consent (Sainio, Lauri, and Eriksson, 2001). Patient ignorance, physical and mental imbalance, patient shyness, patients being treated like objects by nurses and physicians, problems with information dissemination, and the tendency of nurses and physicians to fall into a routine were other reported barriers to patients having a decreased likelihood to participate in decision making (Sainio, Eriksson, and Lauri, 2001). Factors reported to impact on a child's ability to participate in decision making include the child's protest, age, maturity, role of the parents, staff attitudes, time, and alternative solutions to the problem (Runeson et al., 2001).

Disparate factors have been identified with regard to patients' participation in decision making when it comes to end-of-life issues. These include the personality of the patient who is dying, the social network, the availability of alternative forms of care, cultural values, and the degree to which the providers of alternative methods of care support the wishes of the patient and family in the decision-making process (Sahlberg-Blom et al., 2000).

DEFINITION

The AACN Synergy Model definition of *participation in decision making* is the "extent to which the patient and the patient's family engages in decision making in aspect of care" (Curley, 1998). Based on the tenets of the model, a Level 1 patient or family has no capacity for decision making and would need a surrogate. A Level 3 patient and family have limited capacity for decision making and seek advice from others. A Level 5 patient and family can make decisions for themselves. The family is an integral part of the patient and part of the team in terms of health care (Kaplow, 2003; AACN, 2003). Research data support that most patients and families want to be involved in decision making regarding priorities of care. Many choose to take an active part in making decisions. They want to gain as much knowledge as possible about their disease and available treatment options.

Despite lack of data demonstrating benefit of patient participation in decision making, researchers conclude that it is warranted on humane grounds alone and that members of the multidisciplinary health care team should engage patients in decision making in varying degrees based on the patient's willingness and ability to participate (Guadagnoli and Ward, 1998).

CASE STUDY

Mrs. C is a female patient of Asian descent who was diagnosed with colon cancer last year. She is non-English speaking and is unaware of her diagnosis due to cultural preferences expressed by her family. The family refuses to allow an interpreter to speak directly with the patient about her cancer diagnosis. Throughout the course of her initial treatment, Mrs. C believed she had an inflammatory bowel disease that could be cured with this therapy. Mrs. C achieved remission that lasted for 8 months. She now presents with recurrent disease and sepsis and is admitted to the intensive care unit for management of hemodynamic instability.

Mrs. C is successfully treated with vigorous resuscitation and broad spectrum antibiotic coverage. Upon stabilization, the oncologist collaborates with the intensivist regarding Mrs. C's physical readiness for possible enrollment into a clinical trial for treatment of her recurrent disease. Because the only treatment available for Mrs. C is experimental, informed consent is required. The family continues to refuse to disclose Mrs. C's diagnosis to her and does not allow the use of an interpreter. The oncologist wishes to explain the rationale for the therapy, the potential side effects, the risks of therapy, and the symptoms that should be reported. This is unable to be completed without the family's consent. The oncologist and staff are concerned that Mrs. C is participating in the consent process without all the necessary information. They feel that the patient is being deceived and that attainment of optimal outcomes of care is being hampered due to the withholding of information.

By advocating for a patient's right to know and insisting that an interpreter be used to disclose information to Mrs. C about her diagnosis to gain her consent for the experimental therapy, a lack of respect for the cultural aspects impacting care and further distrust for physicians and hospitals will result. The family insists that disclosing the diagnosis to Mrs. C will have a negative impact.

Upon careful consideration, it was agreed that Mrs. C would not be told of her condition but would be told that the treatment was needed for the inflammatory bowel syndrome. All other essential information was given and Mrs. C consented to the experimental therapy.

APPLICATION OF THE CASE STUDY TO THE SYNERGY MODEL

In this case, Mrs. C's family would be considered a Level 5 for decision making. They were able to understand the ramifications of the patient participating in a clinical trial. Mrs. C would be considered a Level 3 for decision making. If she was not competent in this area, she would be considered a Level 1. Although she was mentally, physically, and emotionally competent to render informed consent to participate in the decision-making process, she depended on her family for the information needed to provide consent.

Although it is the obligation of health care providers to assist the patient in decision making by providing relevant information (Beauchamp and Childress, 1994), consideration of other dimensions that impact these decisions deserve equal consideration. In this case, Mrs. C's dignity was maintained and an optimal outcome was achieved.

Mrs. C is vulnerable because of the physical stressors she will be facing in relation to her disease and upcoming treatment. The toxicities associated with her upcoming therapy will likely increase Mrs. C's vulnerability. Her level of resiliency would be considered low, because her remission was short. Mrs. C has a high level of resource availability; she has a very supportive family and she is insured. The pharmaceutical company sponsoring the trial is supporting the cost of the upcoming therapy.

In patients who feel decision making is important, staff should work to enhance opportunities for patients and encourage them to participate in decisions related to their care (Sainio and Lauri, 2003). In the case of children, it is suggested that they be viewed as autonomous and health care providers should promote their participation in decision making (Runeson et al., 2002). Regardless of the patient's age, health care providers should assess the patient's readiness for participation in decision making (Guadagnoli and Ward, 1998) and identify the degree to which patients wish to participate (Barry and Henderson, 1996).

Incorporating patient preferences into treatment decisions is challenging (Roter, 2000), and it takes time and effort to provide them with the information needed to make informed decisions. Approaches to ensure that patients obtain quality information and other forms of support for decision making entails acquiring resources if they are to be well implemented (Entwistle, 2000).

REFERENCES

AACN. (2003). *Characteristics of Patients, Clinical Units and Systems of Concern to Nurse.* Available at: http://www.aacn.org.certcorp/certcorp.nsf/signmodel. Accessed April 26, 2004.

Avis, M. (1994). Choice Cuts: An Exploratory Study of Patients' Views About Participation in Decision-Making in a Day Surgery Unit. *International Journal of Nursing Studies* 31(3): 289–298.

Barry, B., and Henderson, A. (1996). Nature of Decision-Making in the Terminally Ill Patient. *Cancer Nursing* 19(5): 384–391.

Beauchamp, T. L., and Childress, J. F. (1994). *Principles of Biomedical Ethics,* 4th ed. New York: Oxford University Press.

Biley, F. C. (1992). Some Determinants that Affect Patient Participation in Decision-Making About Nursing Care. *Journal of Advanced Nursing* 17(4): 414–421.

Blackwell, L. J., Murphy, S. T., Frank, G., Michel, V., and Azen, S. (1995). Ethnicity and Attitudes Toward Patient Autonomy. *Journal of the American Medical Association* 274(10): 820–825.

Brody, D. S. (1980). The Patient's Role in Clinical Decision-Making. *Annals of Internal Medicine* 93(5): 718–722.

Cahill, J. (1998). Patient Participation—A Review of the Literature. *Journal of Clinical Nursing* 7(2): 119–128.

Curley, M. A. Q. (1998). Patient-Nurse Synergy: Optimizing Patients' Outcomes. *American Journal of Critical Care* 7(1): 64–72.

Davidson, B. J. (1997). Empowerment of Men Newly Diagnosed with Prostate Cancer in Treatment Decision-Making. The University of Manitoba (Canada), doctoral dissertation.

Entwistle, V. A. (2000). Supporting and Resourcing Treatment Decision-Making: Some Policy Considerations. *Health Expectations* 3(1): 77–85.

Gattelari, M., Voigt, K. J., Butow, P. N., and Tattersall, M. H. N. (2002). When the Treatment Goal is Not Cure: Are Cancer Patients Equipped to Make Informed Decisions. *Journal of Clinical Oncology* 20(2): 503–513.

Guadagnoti, E., and Ward, P. (1998). Patient Participation in Decision-Making. *Social Science and Medicine* 47(3): 329–339.

Henderson, A., and Shum, D. (2003). Decision-Making Preferences Towards Surgical Intervention in a Hong Kong Chinese Population. *International Nursing Review* 50(2): 95–100.

Kaplow, R. (2003). AACN Synergy Model for Patient Care: A Framework to Optimize Outcomes." *Critical Care Nurse* 23(Suppl): 27–30.

Kravitz, R. L., and Melnikov, J. (2001). Engaging Patients in Medical Decision Making. *British Medical Journal* 323(7313): 584–585.

Margalith, I., and Shapiro, A. (1997). Anxiety and Patient Participation in Clinical Decision-Making: The Case of Patients with Ureteral Calculi. *Social Science and Medicine* 45(3): 419–427.

Roter, D. (2000). The Medical Visit Context to Treatment Decision-Making and the Therapeutic Relationship. *Health Expectations* 3(1): 17–25.

Runeson, I., Enskär, K., Elander, G., and Hermerén, G. (2001). Professional's Perceptions of Children's Participation in Decision Making in Healthcare. *Journal of Clinical Nursing* 10(1): 70–78.

Runeson, I., Hallstrom, I., Elander, G., and Hermerén, G. (2002). Children's Participation in the Decision-Making Process During Hospitalization: An Observational Study. *Nursing Ethics: An International Journal of Healthcare Professionals* 9(6): 583–598.

Sahlberg-Blom, E., Ternestedt, B., and Johansson, J. (2000). Patient's Participation in Decision Making at the End of Life as Seen by a Close Relative. *Nursing Ethics: An International Journal of Healthcare Professionals* 7(4): 296–313.

Sainio, C., Eriksson, E., and Lauri, S. (2001). Patient Participation in Decision Making About Care: The Cancer Patient's Point of View. *Cancer Nursing* 24(3): 172–179.

Sainio, C., and Lauri, S. (2003). Cancer Patients' Decision-Making Regarding Treatment and Nursing Care. *Journal of Advanced Nursing* 41(3): 250–260.

Sainio, C., Lauri, S., and Eriksson, E. (2001). Cancer Patients' Views and Experiences of Participation in Care and Decision Making. *Nursing Ethics: An International Journal of Healthcare Professionals* 8(2): 97–113.

Sheehan, P. K. (1994). Body Image, Decision-Making, and Breast Cancer Treatment. Boston College, doctoral dissertation.

Shemmings, D. (2000). Professionals' Attitudes to Children's Participation in Decision-Making: A Dichotomous Account and Doctrinal Contests. *Child and Family Social Work* 5(3): 235–243.

Thompson, S. C., Pitts, J. S., and Schwankovsky, L. (1993). Preferences for Involvement in Medical Decision-Making: Situational and Demographic Influences. *Patient Education and Counseling* 22(3): 1335–1340.

CHAPTER 9

PREDICTABILITY

Roberta Kaplow, PhD, RN, CCNS, CCRN

INTRODUCTION

What is the likelihood that a patient will develop a pressure ulcer given the patient's clinical condition? Will the patient be successfully terminated from mechanical ventilation? Will the patient with multiple organ dysfunction syndrome survive? How many nurses will be needed for the next shift? These are just a few questions that health care providers ask themselves or others in an attempt to predict aspects of care.

Health care providers use a range of instruments or prediction models to help answer questions like these. For example, there are a number of valid and reliable instruments available to help predict the likelihood of development of a pressure ulcer and they are based on different clinical indices. Given a patient's general risk, preventative strategies can be implemented to avert pressure ulcer development.

Weaning parameters are often assessed on patients prior to extubation. These, too, are physiologic indices to help health care providers predict whether the patient will tolerate extubation. Though not a predictor for all patients, values obtained may help predict whether reintubation would likely be needed if extubated.

Investigators of studies have reported mortality rates of patients with multiple organ dysfunction syndrome. They cite statistics based on the number of organs that have failed. Other investigators have used acuity systems to predict whether patients will survive an ICU admission.

Nurses are frequently asked to anticipate a critically ill patient's needs for the remainder of a shift and complete patient acuity information. These data are to be used to help predict the number of nurses who will be needed for the upcoming shift.

Given the increased emphasis on patient outcomes, scientists in numerous specialties often develop studies in an attempt to predict outcomes of care. Physiologic response is one outcome used in these studies. In other studies, prediction equations are reported. The following is a review of the literature in which studies were designed to predict various patient outcomes.

Frangolias and Wilcox (2001) found that patients with cystic fibrosis had significant differences between severity of disease and overall distribution of nocturnal oxygen saturation. Specifically, factors including pulmonary function, illness severity score, and two respiratory parameters correlated with nocturnal oxygen saturation levels. The regression equation developed predicted that 91 percent of patients were less likely to desaturate during sleep.

In another study, Croce, Tolley, and Fabian (2003) developed a prediction model for trauma patients in terms of likelihood for the development of ventilator-assisted pneumonia. Factors in the regression equation included the mechanism of injury (penetrating or blunt), the Glasgow Coma Scale score, the presence or absence of a spinal cord injury, the need for emergent laparotomy, the patient's score on an injury severity scale, the amount of blood transfused, and whether the patient required intubation.

Numerous studies have been conducted attempting to predict treatment outcomes. These include monitoring of select physiologic tests or parameters to predict treatment with interferon in patients with hepatitis C viral infection (Beccarello et al., 2002). In another study, investigators reported that weak cytotoxic T-lymphocyte responses found at the end of interferon therapy might predict further relapse of hepatitis C (Amaraa et al., 2003).

In addition to physiologic variables, studies have been developed to predict discharge outcomes. Salbach and colleagues (2001) evaluated whether the gait speed of patients following acute stroke predicted the destination of patients upon hospital discharge. Verbeek and associates (2003) evaluated patients who were survivors of cancer with regard to their occupational rehabilitation processes and their ability to return to work. Hebert and peers (1996) developed a questionnaire to determine the feasibility of predicting functional decline in the elderly living in the community. In this study, six items on the questionnaire were predictors of functional decline.

Grimm and colleagues (2003) evaluated patients with idiopathic dilated cardiomyopathy who had placement of an implantable cardioverter defibrillator. They found that the patients' left ventricular ejection fraction significantly predicted whether these patients would sustain ventricular dysrhythmias. Meldon and peers (2003) evaluated a triage risk screening tool to predict recidivism in the emergency department and hospitalization of elderly patients. They found that the presence of two or more risk factors on the screening tool predicted these two outcome variables.

Other physiologic prediction studies include the use of a questionnaire to predict asthma in adults (Baie et al., 1998); the use of a visual analogue pain scale to predict physical activities, thermal discriminability related to best pain relief, and drug intake (Yang et al., 1991); the use of a multistage filed test to predict peak oxygen consumption (Vanderthommen et al., 2002); the use of electrocardiographic data to predict short-term cardiac outcomes (need for percutaneous coronary intervention or catheterization) (Blomkalns et al., 2003); the use of the International Labour Office radiographic classification to predict arterial oxygen desaturation in patients with asbestosis (Lee et al., 2003); and the effect on mortality with the presence of specific electrocardiographic characteristics and levels of high B-type natriuretic peptide levels on patients with heart failure (Vrtovec et al., 2003).

Other studies have evaluated the ability to predict complications of interventions. These include prediction of the development of stress fractures in males participating in a vigorous exercise program (Shaffer et al., 1999); the 10-year survival rate of patients who undergo total knee replacement procedures (Vazquez-Vela Johnson et al., 2003); and the degree of morbidity and mortality following bone marrow transplantation (Rodrigue et al., 1999).

Prediction of psychosocial outcomes has also been reported in the literature. Meadows, Catalan, and Gazzard (1993) attempted to determine the predictors of a parturient woman's intention to be HIV tested. The strongest predictors of intention included the perceived benefit of the patient, partner, and midwife; the perceived risk of HIV infection; younger age; single status; and poor knowledge of the sexual transmission of the virus. And, finally, in a study of women with the hereditary risk for the development of breast cancer, Loescher (2003) found that younger age and the total symptoms present predicted a higher worry of breast cancer.

Clinical pathways for several conditions have been developed. They have been implemented in many hospitals to enhance efficiency, decrease costs, and improve quality and outcomes of care (Chou and Boldy, 1999). They provide protocols or a template for clinicians to use for suggestions of approaches to care for patients during different phases of an illness. Use of these pathways has resulted in improved health outcomes and decreased length of hospital stay (Chang and Lin, 2003). Based on the knowledge of certain disorders or procedures, patients will likely follow a predicted trajectory. Interventions to help avert problems or have them recognized earlier has led to improved patient outcomes through pathways.

DEFINITION

According to the AACN Synergy Model, *predictability* is a summative characteristic that allows one to expect a certain trajectory (Curley, 1998; AACN, 2003). A Level 1 patient is not predictable, is uncertain, may be an uncommon patient population, or have an uncommon illness or clinical course. The patient does not follow a critical pathway or has a condition for which no clinical pathway has been developed. A Level 3 patient is moderately predictable, is wavering, and is part of an occasionally noted population. A Level 5 patient is highly predictable and is part of a common population. The patient follows an expected course or critical pathway (Kaplow, 2003).

CASE STUDY

JB is a 58-year-old male patient with a medical history significant for two-packs-per-day smoking, hypertension, angina, dyslipidemia, diet-controlled diabetes mellitus, cardiac stent placement to the right anterior descending coronary artery, myocardial infarction, rheumatoid arthritis, and an L4-5 fusion. He is a fisherman by trade. He came to the emergency department with a chief complaint of substernal chest pain radiating to his jaw and down both arms and abdomen that had been intermittently present for the past 3 weeks.

In the emergency department, he was noted to have ST segment elevation and received oxygen via nasal cannula at 4 liters/minute, aspirin, and a nitroglycerin infusion at 20 mcg/min. The chest pain was somewhat relieved by the nitroglycerin (Tridol®) (pain rating decreased from 8 to 3) and the nitroglycerin infusion was increased to 40 mcg/min. He was subsequently admitted to the intensive care unit with a diagnosis of unstable angina.

The angiography revealed total thrombotic occlusion. Angioplasty and restenting were performed and the patient returned to the intensive care unit for postprocedure management. While in the intensive care unit, the nurse, upon speaking with the patient, learned that JB had stopped taking his antiplatelet therapy that had been prescribed for him when he had his initial stent procedure. The nurse also discussed smoking cessation strategies and dietary modifications that were indicated with JB.

The patient had an uneventful course in the intensive care unit and was discharged home on aspirin, simvastatin, ticlopidine, and the NicoDerm® patch. The nurse caring for JB emphasized the importance of adhering to the regimen and provided him with contact information, including signs and symptoms to report and actions to take in the event of future cardiac symptoms.

APPLICATION OF THE CASE STUDY TO THE SYNERGY MODEL

JB presented as a Level 5 in terms of predictability, given his history of unstable angina, stenting of his right anterior descending coronary artery, hypertension, smoking, dyslipidemia, diabetes, and stopping his antiplatelet therapy resulted in coronary stent occlusion. JB had a predictable response to the chest pain management he received. He also had a predictable response to the restenting and postprocedure unfractionated heparin, aspirin, and the glycoprotein IIb/IIIa inhibitor he received.

The nurses caring for JB demonstrated high levels of clinical judgment, collaboration, and clinical inquiry by following the most recent American Heart Association guidelines (www.americanheart.org) for the management of chest pain, allowing JB to ventilate his concerns about his condition and working with other members of the multidisciplinary team. The nurses demonstrated high levels as facilitators of learning when providing patient education regarding the importance of managing potential causes of problems including diet, smoking, and management of hypertension and cholesterol.

In addition, JB exhibited a low level of stability and a high level of vulnerability upon admission. Optimal outcomes were achieved for him during this episode. A clinician's ability to predict outcomes of care can assist in preparing patients and families regarding outcomes and prognosis (Croce et al., 2003).

REFERENCES

AACN. (2003). *Characteristics of Patients, Clinical Units and Systems of Concern to Nurse.* Available at: http://www.aacn.org/certcorp/certcorp.nsf/synmodel. Accessed April 26, 2004.

Amaraa, R., Mareckova, H., Urbanek, P., and Fucikova, T. (2003). Immunological Predictors of Different Responses to Combination Therapy with Interferon Alpha and Ribavirin in Patients with Chronic Hepatitis C. *Journal of Gastroenterology* 38(3): 254–259.

Bai, J., Peat, J. K., Berry, G., Marks, G. B., and Woolcock, A. J. (1998). Questionnaire Items that Predict Asthma and Other Respiratory Conditions in Adults. *Chest* 114(5): 1343–1348.

Beccarello, A., Bortolato, L., Triches, C., Paleari, C., Awasum, M. C., Zalunardo, B., Orlando, R., and Lirussi, F. (2002). Monoethylglycin Exylide Kinetics and Galactose Elimination Capacity During Treatment with Interferon-Alfa for Hepatitis C Virus Infection: Possible Predictors of Response. *Current Therapeutic Research, Clinical and Experimental* 63(11): 772–786.

Blomkalns, A. L., Lindsell, C. J., Chandra, A., Osterlund, M. E., Gibler, W. B., Pollack, C. V., Tiffany, B. R., Hollander, J. E., and Hoekstra, J. W. (2003). Can Electrocardiographic Criteria Predict Adverse Cardiac Events and Positive Cardiac Markers? *Academic Emergency Medicine* 10(3): 205–210.

Chang, W., and Lin, C. (2003). A Clinical Pathway for Laparoscopically Assisted Vaginal Hysterectomy: Impact on Costs and Clinical Outcome. *Journal of Reproductive Medicine* 48(4): 247–251.

Chou, S., and Boldy, D. (1999). Patient Perceived Quality-of-Care in Hospitals in the Context of Clinical Pathways: Development of an Approach. *Journal of Evaluation in Clinical Practice* 19(2): 89–93.

Croce, M. A., Tolley, E. A., and Fabianm, T. C. (2003). A Formula for Prediction of Post-Traumatic Pneumonia Based on Early Anatomic and Physiologic Parameters . . . Includes Discussion. *Journal of Trauma-Injury Infection and Critical Care* 54(4): 724–730.

Curley, M. A. Q. (1998). Patient-Nurse Synergy: Optimizing Patients' Outcomes. *American Journal of Critical Care* 7(1): 64–72.

Frangolias, D. D., and Wilcox, P. G. (2001). Predictability of Oxygen Desaturation During Sleep in Patients with Cystic Fibrosis: Clinical, Spirometric, and Exercise Parameters. *Chest* 119(2): 434–441.

Grimm, W., Herzum, I., Muller, H., and Christ, M. (2003). Value of Heart Rate Variability to Predict Ventricular Arrhythmias in Recipients of Prophylactic Defibrillators with Idiopathic Dilated Cardiomyopathy. *Pacing and Clinical Electrophyisology* 26(1): 411–415.

Hebert, R., Bravo, G., Korner-Bitensky, N., and Voyer, L. (1996). Predictive Validity of a Postal Questionnaire for Screening Community-Dwelling Elderly Individuals at Risk for Functional Decline. *Age Ageing* 25(2): 159–167.

Kaplow, R. (2003). AACN Synergy Model for Patient Care: A Framework to Optimize Outcomes. *Critical Care Nurse* 23(Suppl): 27–30.

Lee, Y. C. G., Singh, B., Pang, S. C., deKlerk, W. H., Hillman, D. R., and Musk, A. W. (2003). Radiographic (ILO) Readings Predict Arterial Oxygen Desaturation During Exercise in Subjects with Asbestosis. *Occupational and Environmental Medicine* 60(3): 201–206.

Loescher, L. J. (2003). Cancer Worry in Women with Hereditary Risk Factors for Breast Cancer. *Oncology Nursing Forum* 30(5): 767–772.

Meadows, J., Catalan, J., and Gazzard, B. (1993). 'I Plan to Have the HIV Test'— Predictors of Testing Intention in Women Attending a London Antenatal Clinic. *Academic Emergency Medicine* 10(3): 224–232.

Meldon, S. W., Mion, L. C., Palmer, R. M., Drew, B. L., Connor, J. T., Lewicki, L. J., Bass, D. M., and Emerman, C. L. (2003). A Brief Risk-Stratification Tool to Predict Repeat Emergency Department Visits and Hospitalizations in Older Patients Discharged from the Emergency Department. *Academic Emergency Medicine* 10(3): 224–232.

Rodrigue, J. R., Pearman, T. P., and Moreb, J. (1999). Morbidity and Mortality Following Bone Marrow Transplantation: Predictive Utility of Pre-BMT Affective Functioning, Compliance, and Social Support Stability. *International Journal of Behavioral Medicine* 6(3): 241–254.

Salbach, N. M., Mayo, N. E., Higgins, J., Ahmed, S., Finch, L., Richards, E. (2001). Responsiveness and Predictability of Gait Speed and Other Disability Measures in Acute Stroke. *Archives of Physical Medicine and Rehabilitation* 82(9): 1204–1212.

Shaffer, R. A., Brodine, S. K., Almeida, S. A., Williams, K. M., and Ronaghy, S. (1999). Use of Simple Measures of Physical Activity to Predict Stress Fractures in Young Men Undergoing a Rigorous Physical Training Program. *American Journal of Epidemiology* 149(3): 236–242.

Vanderthommen, M., Fancaux, M., Colinet, C., Lehance, C., Lhermerout, C., Crielaard, J., and Theisen, D. (2002). A Multistage Field Test of Wheelchair Users for Evaluation of Fitness and Prediction of Peak Oxygen Consumption. *Journal of Rehabilitation Research and Development* 39(6): 685–692.

Vazquez-Vela Johnson, G., Worland, R. L., Kennan, J., and Norambuena, N. (2003). Patient Demographics as a Predictor of the Ten-Year Survival Rate in Primary Total Knee Replacement. *Journal of Bone and Joint Surgery—British Volume* 853(1): 52–56.

Verbeek, J., Spelten, E., Kammeijer, M., and Sprangers, M. (2003). Return to Work of Cancer Survivors: A Prospective Cohort Study into the Quality of Rehabilitation by Occupational Physicians. *Occupational and Environmental Medicine* 60(5): 352–357.

Vrtovec, B., Delgado, R., Zewail, A., Thomas, C. D., Richartz, B. M., and Radovancevic, B. (2003). Prolonged QTc Interval and High B-Type Natriuretic Peptide Levels Together Predict Mortality in Patients with Advanced Heart Failure. *Circulation* 107(13): 1764–1769.

Yang, J. C., Clark, W. C., and Janal, M. N. (1991). Sensory Decision Theory and Visual Analogue Scale Indices Predict Status of Chronic Pain Patients Six Months Later. *Journal of Pain and Symptom Management* 6(2): 58–64.

SECTION III

NURSE CHARACTERISTICS

CHAPTER 10

CLINICAL JUDGMENT

Sonya R. Hardin, PhD, RN, CCRN, APRN
Daphne Stannard, PhD, RN, CCRN, CCNS

INTRODUCTION

Clinical judgment is at the heart of nursing. Nurses are both responsible and accountable for making the right decisions at the right moments in time to ensure optimal patient and family outcomes and safe passage through the health care system. There is an art and science to making decisions for and with the patient. Nurses use reflection and critical thinking as they make the best decision for the patient given the context of the situation. Clinical judgment emerges as a competency that has historically been grounded in the nursing process of assessment, planning, intervention, and evaluation. Often clinical judgment is replaced by ritual and tradition or policies and procedures. It has been shown that novice and expert nurses used different thinking processes. Novice nurses used the nursing process while expert nurses relied on experience, intuition, practical intelligence, and academic knowledge (Benner, 2001; Benner et al., 1996).

CLINICAL JUDGMENT

Understanding the nursing process of various diseases requires the ability to utilize clinical judgment in all phases of assessing, planning, intervening, and evaluating the plan of care for patients and families. The steps in the nursing process are utilized as a method for problem solving that leads to appropriate clinical judgment. A form of critical thinking, the nursing process, is considered to be a logical and rational way for nurses to organize and manage care. In the assessment phase, the nurse encounters or recognizes a problem. The data are collected through objective and subjective methods and a nursing diagnosis or a conclusion is reached. Nursing assessment includes being competent to collect a medical history and to discern the specific cues that are pertinent to the patient's signs and symptoms. The nurse should gather physical, psychosocial, cultural, developmental, and spiritual data. Data are analyzed in a comparative nature with the expected and unexpected nature of the disease process.

Planning begins with identification of patient goals. These guide the selection of interventions. At that point, a plan of action is developed based upon the hypothesis of potential reasons for the problem. Testing of the hypothesis occurs as the nurse utilizes different interventions to improve patient outcomes. Implementation involves the delivery of specific interventions while continually reassessing the patient's response. The interventions are continuously being evaluated as the nurse monitors the response of the patient. The evaluation phase includes the nurse examining the patient's progress, evaluating patient outcomes, and revising the plan of care given patient response. Throughout the nursing process, various critical thinking skills are utilized such as distinguishing relevant data from the irrelevant, recognizing patterns and relationships in the data, determining the patient's desired outcomes, utilizing knowledge to perform interventions, and comparing the patient's response in relation to the desired outcomes.

Expert Clinical Judgment

Expert clinicians utilize intuition, reflection, and methods that allow the nurse to truly know the patient. Intuition is a "way of knowing where facts are felt directly rather than arrived at in a linear manner" (Rew, 1996, p. 149). According to Benner (2001), the expert does not rely only on analytic rules for making clinical judgment but uses an intuitive grasp, which is a deep understanding of the total situation. Reflection is a process of thinking about a situation in relationship to previous experiences. Establishing meaningful connections between experiences is an aspect of reflection. A comparative analysis and reframing of the situation is thought through as the practitioner comes to integrate experiences into the present moment. Lastly, expert clinical judgment involves knowing the patient as a person and through individual patterns of response. Understanding of the patient occurs when the nurse can see the "big picture." This comes about through being with the patient, listening, sensing, and experiencing the nuances of the individual.

The advanced practice nurse provides clinical expertise in solving patient problems and in developing complex plans of care based upon the needs of the patient (Moloney-Harmon, 1999). An expert nurse synthesizes, interprets, and makes decisions based on complex, sometimes conflicting, sources of data for the patient. Clinical judgment is displayed by developing, implementing, and evaluating research-based algorithms, decision trees, protocols, and care plans for patients and patient populations. Clinical judgment is role modeled for the staff as the expert nurse provides direct patient care, develops educational programs, and evaluates practice (Moloney-Harmon, 1999).

Competency for Evaluating Clinical Judgment

Nine competencies have been identified by Alfaro-LeFevre (1999) for clinical judgment and are outlined as .follows. Nurses demonstrating clinical judgment use references, the nursing process, and resources. Assessments are performed and priorities are set systematically. Nursing actions are only performed when indications for the action are understood. Nurses should have knowledge of standards of care and follow the policies and procedures established by the organization in the delivery of care. Patient-centered care should be delivered through an understanding of the patient. Nurses should know how to use patient technology to ensure safe care.

The nurse should display competency in the recognition of assessment data and the analysis of objective and subjective data. An awareness of one's ability and limitations, the ability to identify patient needs, and the need to set goals with the patient are all competencies for clinical judgment (AACN, 2003b).

DEFINITION

Clinical judgment is defined as the use of clinical reasoning including decision making, critical thinking, and the global grasp of a situation, coupled with nursing skills acquired through a process of integrating education, experimental knowledge, and evidenced-based guidelines (AACN, 2002).

Clinical judgment qualitatively differs depending on where one is located along the skill-acquisition continuum. A central finding of Benner and colleagues' research (1996) is that nurses at different stages of skill acquisition live in different clinical worlds. Change, not the mere passage of time, is the defining characteristic of experience. As one gains experience in practice, one's clinical judgment is further honed. As such, clinical judgment can range from deliberate, conscious decision making that is characteristic of nurses at the competent stage of skill acquisition (or Level 3 nurses) to a more holistic understanding and response-based practice typical of expert (or Level 5) nurses.

The advanced-beginner level of skill acquisition is a time of active clinical learning and focusing on mastering technical skills. Nurses at this stage (or Level 1 nurses) are capable of collecting and interpreting basic level data. Clinical decisions, however, are limited to the new nurse's knowledge. Thus, newer nurses frequently "delegate up" to more seasoned health care providers who essentially share their clinical judgment with the newer nurses (Benner et al., 1996). Examples of delegating up that are commonly seen surround clinical issues such as giving PRN medications, ordering extra laboratory tests, changing the frequency of documenting vital signs, or when to notify the physician. As nurses acquire more experience, they rely less on the clinical judgments of others.

At the competent stage of skill acquisition (Level 3), nurses have improved organizational ability and have mastered many technical skills. As such, nurses at this stage are more focused on managing the patient's condition. The clinical world of this nurse is organized by planning for and anticipating likely events in the clinical situation (Benner et al., 1996). Nurses at this stage still seek guidance from more seasoned clinicians when they are puzzled with the clinical picture or when confronted with something new. Nurses at the competent stage of skill acquisition, however, can readily care for usual and customary patients using their hard-won experiential knowledge.

Expert practice (Level 5) is characterized by an increased ability to recognize whole patterns and a developed sense of salience where relevant clinical aspects simply stand out for the nurse without recourse to conscious deliberation (Benner et al., 1996). The expert nurse can synthesize and interpret multiple, often conflicting, sources of data. Understanding the unique needs of the patient and family situation and responding in a fluid, almost seamless fashion, is the hallmark of response-based expert practice.

CASE STUDY

HS was a 45-year-old female admitted for bariatric surgery. She weighed 280 pounds and had a history of smoking, headaches, depression, hypercholesterolemia, and an appendectomy and removal of a spleen as a result of blunt trauma in a vehicular accident. She was admitted to the ICU postoperatively due to complications associated with a modified laparoscopic minigastric bypass. Given adhesions from the previous removal of her spleen, nine laparoscopic puncture sites were required.

During the surgery, the colon was lacerated, resulting in the need for a repair. HS had a number 20 angiocath in the right hand with D5½ normal saline running at 125 cc/hr. She was NPO with a nasogastric tube connected to low wall suction and was receiving oxygen via a nasal cannula at 4 liters/min. HS had a midline incision with a dressing held in place by Montgomery straps. She was wearing TED hose and a sequential compression device. A catheter to straight drainage had dark concentrated urine. Her hemoglobin was 8.8 g/dl and the oxygen saturation had been running at 88 percent.

The nurse caring for the patient identified the following nursing diagnoses: alternation in ventilation associated with a history of smoking and postoperative status, potential for infection associated with postoperative status, and hypovolemia associated with postoperative status. Nursing interventions included teaching the patient the importance of coughing and deep breathing and the use of the incentive spirometer. The nurse knew to monitor intake and output, vital signs, and EKG.

Upon the initial assessment of the patient, the nurse identified diminished breath sounds in the right lower lobe, oxygen saturation of 68 percent, shortness of breath, anxiety, and confusion (oriented to name only). The nurse observed the following: abdomen firm, no audible bowel sounds, abdominal dressing dry and intact, pedal pulses present, 1+ pitting edema in her ankles, and cardiac monitor showed sinus tachycardia at a rate of 112, B/P 110/64, and a respiratory rate of 44.

The nurse contacted the physician and provided an update on the patient's condition that focused on the patient's respiratory status and low urinary output. Orders were received to give 40 mg of furosemide (Lasix®) IV and 100 percent non-rebreather mask. The Lasix® was administered with minimal response and the oxygen saturation increased to 78 percent. The nurse called the physician back after 30 minutes and informed him that the patient's oxygen saturation was still in the 70s and that the patient's respiratory rate was 40–44. Orders were received for a ventilation and perfusion scan. Results of the scan showed scatter microemboli throughout the lower right lobe. The patient was placed on BiPAP with a resulting oxygen saturation of 88 percent. The head of the bed was raised to a 90-degree angle and ongoing monitoring was continued.

APPLICATION OF THE CASE STUDY TO THE SYNERGY MODEL

The nurse realized that this bariatric patient was at risk for pulmonary emboli. The signs and symptoms of pulmonary embolus were recognized and interventions for this patient included calling the physician, vigilant monitoring and reassessing the patient, administering medication, and ordering diagnostic tests. The nurse in this case was working at a Level 3 with respect to clinical judgment by sorting out extraneous details from the patterns and trends that predicted the direction of pulmonary embolus. The Level 3 nurse should compare the patient's responses to desired outcomes through the knowledge of anatomy and physiology, invasive and noninvasive diagnostic studies, relevant pharmacology, signs and symptoms, and patient care management for disease processes.

The nurse at the Level 1 of clinical judgment is capable of collecting and interpreting basic level data. Algorithms, decision trees, and protocols are utilized as analytical tools for decision making with all populations. The Level 1 nurse matches formal knowledge and clinical events in formulating basic care decisions. At Level 1, expected outcomes are recognized and clinical decisions are limited to one's ability. The nurse will defer to expert clinicians when difficult situations arise (Curley, 1998; Kaplow, 2003).

A Level 3 nurse collects and interprets complex patient data while focusing on key elements of the case. The ability to sort out extraneous details from the patterns and trends that predict the direction of the illness is performed at this level. The nurse follows algorithms, decision trees, and protocols, yet is comfortable deviating from them with patient populations who have been cared for in the past (Curley, 1998; Kaplow, 2003).

The nurse at Level 5 will synthesize and interpret multiple, sometimes conflicting, sources of data. Decisions are based on an immediate grasp of the whole picture unless working with a new patient population. The Level 5 nurse uses past experiences to anticipate potential problems. Unexpected outcomes are anticipated and an understanding of collaboration with multidisciplinary personnel is appreciated as a plan of care is designed. The nurse has skill in delegating others to act on behalf of the patient and family.

Clinical judgment is a culmination of knowledge and the ability to differentiate the expected from the unexpected response of the patient from nursing and medical interventions (AACN, 2003a). Being able to integrate knowledge and understand the impact of multisystem influences on the patient and family is central to clinical judgment. Using the nursing process to frame the practice of nursing in the delivery of care is essential to ensure safe passage of the patient through the current health care systems.

REFERENCES

AACN. (2002). *Competency Level Descriptors for Nurse Characteristics*. Aliso Viejo, CA: AACN Certification Corporation.

AACN. (2003a). *CCRN Certification Blue Print for Study*. Aliso Viejo, CA: American Association of Critical Care Nurses.

AACN. (2003b). *Survey of Critical Care Nursing Practice*. Aliso Viejo, CA: American Association of Critical Care Nurses.

Alfaro-LeFevre, R. (1999). *Critical Thinking in Nursing: A Practical Approach*, 2nd ed. Philadelphia: W.B. Saunders.

Benner, P. A. (2001). *From Novice to Expert*. Upper Saddle River, NJ: Prentice Health Hall.

Benner, P. A., Tanner, C. A., and Chelsa, C. A. (1996). *Expertise in Nursing Practice: Caring, Clinical Judgment, and Ethics*. New York: Springer.

Curley, M. A. Q. (1998). Patient-Nurse Synergy: Optimizing Patients' Outcomes. *American Journal of Critical Care* 7(1): 64–72.

Kaplow, R. (2003). AACN Synergy Model for Patient Care: A Framework to Optimize Outcomes. *Critical Care Nurse* 23 (1, Suppl): 27–30.

Moloney-Harmon, P. A. (1999). The Synergy Model: Contemporary Practice of the Clinical Nurse Specialist. *Critical Care Nurse* 19(2): 101–104.

Rew, L. (1996). *Awareness in Healing*. Albany, NY: Delmar.

CHAPTER 11

ADVOCACY/MORAL AGENCY

Daphne Stannard, PhD, RN, CCRN, CCNS
Sonya R. Hardin, PhD, RN, CCRN, APRN

CvP A 804

INTRODUCTION

Serving as an advocate for a patient, family member, or another health care provider is commonly understood as working on behalf of another. Although nurses typically serve as advocates across settings and patient populations, nowhere is advocacy more evident than in critical care arenas. Critically ill patients are vulnerable and often incapacitated, while their loved ones are usually stunned and anxious by the gravity of the situation.

Critical care nurses are confronted daily with situations that require them to act on their patient's behalf. Many state practice acts include being an advocate in their bylaws. According to the American Nurses Association, the nurse will "advocate for and strive to protect the health, safety, and rights of their patients" (Fowler and Benner, 2001, p. 434). To optimize patient outcomes, it is important to understand what advocacy means as it relates to nursing.

Patient advocacy continues to receive attention within the nursing literature. The values of nursing are often associated with commitment, caring, compassion, integrity, competence, spirit of inquiry, confidentiality, responsibility, values-based decision making, and respect for the person (International Council of Nurses, 2000; Tschudin, 1999). Advocacy occurs when a nurse protects the patient's human and legal rights (American Nurses Association, 1987; Craven and Hirnle, 2000; Ersoy and Altun, 1997; International Council of Nurses, 2000).

Advocacy has become an ethical obligation for the nurse to work for the patients and family when a real or potential ethical problem exists. Patients and families are in vulnerable positions within the health care system and need nurses to advocate for them when they cannot speak for themselves or when others do not hear their voices (Davis et al., 2003). Nurses must be prepared to advocate for clients through the delivery of care.

The role of patient advocacy has been explored by both Japanese and Turkish nurses (Davis et al., 2003; Altun and Ersoy, 2003). A search of the Japanese literature found that the rights to informed consent, refuse treatment, know a diagnosis and prognosis, be treated with dignity, and privacy were the major themes. Japanese values of advocacy include "belongingness," freedom, empathy, dependency, and reciprocity due to their focus on smooth and pleasant social relationships (Davis et al., 2003). Davis and colleagues (2003) conducted a research study of 24 nurses' views of advocacy. The findings suggest that Japanese nurses believe that they should advocate for patients because nurses have the closest contact with patients and a responsibility exists to provide holistic health.

A Turkish longitudinal nursing study focused on nursing students' perspectives of patient rights and their attitudes during their educational program. Findings included students' beliefs that euthanasia should be allowed in accordance with patient wishes. Over time, students increased their belief that patients should know their diagnosis. One third of the students believed that severely disabled newborn babies should be allowed to die. The researchers believe that instruction in ethics in nursing education is needed (Altun and Ersoy, 2003). Both the Japanese and the Turkish nursing studies conclude that awareness and sensitivity to advocacy is needed in the delivery of care.

Competency of Advocacy

Competency is displayed when the nurse advocates for the patient and family regardless of personal values. Ethical or moral decisions are based on supporting the rights of the patient. The nurse supports and advocates for resolutions with the patient, family, and colleagues in ethical and clinical issues (AACN, 2003b). Advocacy can take many forms; however, ultimately it is the nurse working in the best interest of the patient.

DEFINITION

When researching the term advocacy, many definitions were found. According to *Merriam-Webster Dictionary* (1998), the word *advocacy* means "an argument or pleading for a cause or proposal." The *Random House Dictionary* (1990) definition correlates with the previous but also includes, "espousing or taking up support by argument." A third reference, *The American Heritage Dictionary of the English Language* (2000) defines advocacy as "pleading or arguing in favor of something such as a cause, idea, or policy." In addition, AACN has defined advocacy as "respecting and supporting the basic values, rights, and benefits of the critically ill patients" (Thelan et al., 1998, p. 29). The AACN further defines advocacy by stating that nurse advocates will respect and support the right of the patient or patient's designated surrogate to autonomous informed decision making; intervene when the best interest of the patient is in question; help the patient to obtain necessary care; provide education and support to help the patient or the patient's designated surrogate make decisions; represent the patient in accordance with the patient's choices; support the decisions of the patient or the patient's designated surrogate; intercede for patients who cannot speak for themselves in situations that require immediate action; monitor and safeguard the quality of care that the patients receive; and act as a liaison between the patient, patient's family, and other health care professionals (Thelan et al., 1998).

Advocacy can be defined as active support. As such, advocacy is just one aspect of moral agency. Advocacy is discussed frequently in the nursing literature, which is perhaps why more nurses feel comfortable thinking of themselves as advocates rather than as moral agents. However, by serving as an advocate, one is expressing one's agency. Put another way, a nurse's agency can be described in many ways, and when he or she acts as an advocate, then agency is characterized as advocacy. Simply stated, moral agency connotes understanding and action and advocacy connotes support.

Agency is a term borrowed from ethics that refers to the openness, recognition of, and willingness to act on matters of significance (Beauchamp and Childress, 2001; Taylor, 1985). All human beings have agency and, therefore, all human beings are agents. How particular human beings understand themselves and the effect they have in any given situation, however, influences one's sense of agency. Agency at the different stages of skill acquisition is related to the contributions a nurse can make at a given stage of skill acquisition. Thus, while all nurses are agents, their sense of agency differs depending on where they are along the skill acquisition continuum (Benner, 1984).

Moral agency refers to one's ability to act upon or influence a situation and can be understood as how a critical care nurse, for instance, engages, responds, and changes a clinical situation on behalf of critically ill patients, their family members, and other members of the health care team. As clinical agents, advanced beginners (or Level 1 nurses) attempt to manage patient care according to specified orders and plans of care (Benner et al., 1996). At the competent stage of skill acquisition (Level 3 nurses), agency shows up as one's ability to plan and order the clinical priorities of patient and family care. Expert nurses (or Level 5 nurses) have expert moral agency. The development of clinical expertise inherently demands the development of ethical expertise (Benner et al., 1996). Thus, expert nurses are fully able and willing to take a stand on what they believe is important in a situation and can provide moral and clinical action that is based on what is required in the situation by the patient or family member. Action that is based on what the other desires and requires can also be called *response-based action*. The hallmark of expertise is a response-based practice (Benner et al., 1999).

More recently, the Synergy Model, developed by the AACN, defines advocacy as "working on another's behalf and representing the concerns of the patient" (AACN, 2003a, p. 26). Advocacy is serving as a moral agent in identifying and helping to resolve ethical and clinical concerns within and outside the clinical setting (AACN, 2003a). Lastly, advocacy is a process that helps patients to access appropriate health care resources. It protects the patient's rights to select values that sustain life, exercise personal judgment, and make decisions without coercion (Thelan et al., 1998).

Based upon the tenets of the AACN Synergy Model, a nurse at a Level 1 competency works on behalf of the patient and begins to self-assess personal values.

The nurse is aware of the patient's rights and ethical conflicts that may surface during care of the patient. Ethical or moral decisions are made based upon guiding principles and nurses' personal values. The nurse works as an advocate when a patient's framework is consistent with their values.

A Level 1 nurse is aware of death as an outcome and works on behalf of the patient through rule-based clinical decisions. A Level 3 nurse considers the patient's values and incorporates these values into the care, even if these values differ from their own. The nurse is aware of and works for the rights of the patient and family. Moral decision making can deviate from the rules during the delivery of care. A Level 3 nurse can be flexible in allowing the patient or family to represent themselves whenever possible and can identify internal resources for the patient and family when complex decisions are required in providing care. Level 5 nurses are capable of advocating for the patient, family, and community no matter if their personal values are congruent with the client. The nurse advocates for resolution of ethical conflicts through the utilization of internal and external resources. A Level 5 nurse empowers the patient and family to drive moral decision making through a mutuality of relationships with providers (AACN, 2002).

CASE STUDY

Mr. B. was admitted to the intensive care unit from the operating room after emergent cardiac surgery. He was on the ventilator, sedated, and had marginally stable vital signs. The nurse noted that his chest tube had drained 1800 ml. A STAT hemoglobin showed a result of 6.2 g/dL. The physician ordered a transfusion of three units of packed red blood cells to be given as soon as possible. While looking for the patient's informed consent for blood transfusions, the nurse noted that the patient was listed as a Jehovah's Witness. The nurse verified with the significant other that the patient indeed was a practicing Jehovah's Witness. Having knowledge of the patient's beliefs, the nurse immediately called the physician and obtained an order for continuous circuit auto transfusion. The order to give packed red blood cells was cancelled.

APPLICATION OF THE CASE STUDY TO THE SYNERGY MODEL

Jehovah's Witnesses are members of the Watch Tower Bible and Tract Society, a religious denomination founded in the United States in 1872. There are approximately 6 million Jehovah's Witnesses worldwide (Marsh and Bevan, 2002). Between 1961 and 2000, any Jehovah's Witness transfused with a blood product would have been expelled from the Society, a policy known as "disfellowship." Disfellowship was abandoned in the year 2000; however, rejection of blood products is self-inflicted.

There are strong ethical reasons to accede and adapt to the wishes and beliefs of the patient. Nurses must ensure that Jehovah's Witnesses are asked to decide which blood products are acceptable and then support their decision (Marsh and Bevan, 2002).

Understanding the patient's rights is essential to ensuring advocacy. Patients are often incapable of voicing their wants or needs due to being in crisis. Ethically and legally, nurses are expected to act in the best interest of the patient. In this example, the patient was on a ventilator and sedated and was not capable of making his wishes known to the staff. The nurse acted as an advocate by finding a mechanism by which the patient's values and the values of western medicine could be honored. This nurse was acting at Level 5. At Level 5, the nurse works toward resolving an ethical dilemma in such a manner that the patient's perspective is valued. The nurse recognized that the right of the patient had to drive the decision regarding volume replacement.

The core concept behind the AACN Synergy Model is that the unique needs or characteristics of patients and their families influence and drive the characteristics or competencies of nurses (Biel, 1997). According to the model, optimal patient outcomes result when patients' and nurses' characteristics are matched (Curley, 1998). The process of matching the needs and characteristics of a particular patient and family with those of the nurse creates synergy or the cooperative activity of two or more agents or people, which, when working together, produce a combined result greater than they would have if working alone (Stannard, 1999). Advocacy and moral agency are critical components for nurses practicing in all settings and at all stages of skill acquisition.

REFERENCES

AACN. (2002). *Competency Level Descriptors for Nurse Characteristics*. Aliso Viejo, CA: AACN Certification Corporation.

AACN. (2003a). *CCRN Certification Blue Print for Study*. Aliso Viejo, CA: American Association of Critical Care Nurses.

AACN. (2003b). *Survey of Critical Care Nursing Practice*. Aliso Viejo, CA: American Association of Critical Care Nurses.

Altun, I., and Ersoy, N. (2003). Undertaking the Role of Patient Advocate: A Longitudinal Study of Nursing Students. *Nursing Ethics* 10(5): 462–471.

American Heritage Dictionary of the English Language, The. (2000). Boston, MA: American Heritage.

American Nurses Association. (1987). *Code for Nurses with Interpretive Statements*. Washington, DC: ANA.

Beauchamp, T., and Childress, J. (2001). *Principles of Biomedical Ethics*, 5th ed. New York: Oxford.

Benner, P. (1984). *From Novice to Expert: Excellence and Power in Clinical Nursing Practice*. Menlo Park, CA: Addison-Wesley.

Benner, P., Hooper-Kyriakidis, P., and Stannard, D. (1999). *Clinical Wisdom and Interventions in Critical Care: A Thinking-in-Action Approach*. Philadelphia: Saunders.

Benner, P., Tanner, C., and Chelsa, C. (1996). *Expertise in Nursing Practice: Caring, Clinical Judgment, and Ethics*. New York: Springer.

Biel, M. (1997). *Reconceptualizing Certified Practice: Envisioning Critical Care Practice of the Future*. Aliso Viejo, CA: AACN Certification Corporation.

Craven, R. F., and Hirnle, C. J. (2000). *Fundamental of Nursing: Human Health and Function*, 4th ed. Philadelphia: Lippincott.

Curley, M. A. Q. (1998). Patient-Nurse Synergy: Optimizing Patients' Outcomes. *American Journal of Critical Care* 7(1): 64–72.

Davis, A. J., Konishi, E., and Tashiro, M. (2003). A Pilot Study of Selected Japanese Nurses' Ideas on Patient Advocacy. *Nursing Ethics* 10(4): 404–413.

Ersoy, N., and Altun, I. (1997). Tendency of Nurses to Undertake the Role of Patient Advocate. *Eubios J Asian International Bioethics* 7: 167–169.

Fowler, M. D., and Benner, P. (2001). Implementing the New Code of Ethics for Nurses: An Interview with Marsha Fowler. *American Journal of Critical Care Nursing* 10(6): 434–437.

International Council of Nurses. (2000). *Code of Ethics for Nurses*. Geneva: ICN.

Merriam-Webster Dictionary. (1998). Springfield, MA: Merriam-Webster.

Moloney-Harmon, P. (1999). The Synergy Model: Contemporary Practice of the Clinical Nurse Specialist. *Critical Care Nurse* 19(2): 101–104.

Marsh, J., and Bevan, D. H. (2002). Haematological care of the Jehovah's Witness Patient. *British Journal of Haematology* 119: 25–37.

Random House Dictionary of English Language. (1990). New York: Random House, Inc.

Stannard, D. (1999). Being a Good Dance Partner: The Synergy Model in Practice. *Critical Care Nurse* 19(6): 86–87.

Taylor, C. (1985). *Philosophical Papers: Human Agency and Language* (vol. 1). New York: Cambridge.

Thelan, L., Urden, L., Lough, M., and Stacy, K. (1998). *Critical Care Nursing: Diagnosis and Treatment*, 3rd ed. St. Louis, MO: Mosby, Inc.

Tschudin, V. (1999). *Nurses Matter: Reclaiming Our Professional Identity*. London: Macmillian.

CHAPTER 12

CARING PRACTICES

Sonya R. Hardin, PhD, RN, CCRN, APRN

INTRODUCTION

Caring is an interactive process between the patient and the nurse that allows each to grow, actualize, and transform toward higher levels of being in the world. A conscious intention to care for patients potentates healing and wholeness (Blattner, 1981). Caring does not discard conventional science and all that medical curing, modern nursing, and medical practices have achieved. The critical care nurse must look beyond the external disease and its treatment by conventional means. Caring requires looking for a deeper source of inner healing that involves a commitment to a particular purpose, which is the protection, enhancement, and preservation of dignity; humanity wholeness; and inner harmony (Blattner, 1981). The nurse caring and the person being cared for are transformed in the process of caring (Watson, 2001).

CARING PRACTICES

Few studies exist that describe caring behaviors in critical care. Burfitt and colleagues (1993) conducted a phenomenological study to describe patients' perceptions of caring exhibited by professional nurses. Caring in critical care units was viewed by patients as attentive, vigilant behavior on the part of the nurses. This vigilance included nurturance and incorporates highly skilled, technical practices as well as basic nursing care.

Caring is a mutual process in which intentions are joined to form a shared experience between the nurse and the patient. An outcome of caring that might be elusive is healing (Burfitt et al., 1993).

CARING SKILLS

Specific skills have been identified in the literature as reflective of caring. Specifically, Patterson and Zderad (1976) and Watson (2001) have categorized activities that represent caring behaviors by the nurse. Patterson and Zderad (1976) recommend that nurses recognize the patient by name. Using the patient's name frequently ensures that the nurse has internalized the person's identity as a human being. Such actions reflect dignity and worth of the person. Nurses should give as much honest information as possible to ensure the patient's understanding of his or her condition as well as recognize that individuals have the right to choose. Acceptance of the patient's feelings and choices is a caring skill that can be acted out authentically through staying with or doing for the patient and family. Nurses should be alert to the patient responses. Patient's responses reflect past experiences and patterns that should be cues to the nurse to therapeutically intervene. Therapeutic interventions executed correctly are typically viewed as caring by patients. Therefore, the nurse's level of competency is an aspect of caring.

Watson (2001) describes 10 clinical "caritas" processes that can be utilized to develop a transpersonal caring relationship. These *caritas* mean acts that are unique and require special attention to carry out. In essence, these 10 caritas describe an authentic caring presence. A caring presence occurs when the nurse actively listens, provides an unconditional positive regard and nonjudgmental stance toward the patient, and creatively uses self and all the ways of knowing to engage in healing practices. Nurses must be genuinely engaged in assisting with basic needs, sustaining a helping-trusting relationship, and being open to others with sensitivity and compassion.

CARING IN NURSING

Milton Mayeroff (1971) describes the ingredients of caring as knowing, alternating rhythms, patience, honesty, trust, humility, hope, and courage. Knowing involves explicit and implicit knowing. Explicit knowing is being able to articulate information while implicit knowing is sensing information that one is unable to express verbally. Knowing a person in a caring relationship means acknowledging the person's strengths and weaknesses while understanding their needs. Alternating rhythms is a term Mayeroff uses to describe the ability to take different viewpoints on a problem and to use a broader point of view. The nurse should demonstrate patience in allowing themselves and clients to grow in their own way. Clients must be allowed to set their own goals and make decisions. Patience is allowing an elderly person the time to slowly walk to the bathroom instead of using a bedpan. Honesty is sincerity in regard to the client's feelings and what they are saying. Being present to the client is a form of honesty to the moment. Humility is an understanding that the care provided is not privileged and that others have the ability to care. Trust is the ability to take a risk into the unknown with a client. Patients need to feel trust in the one who is providing care. Providing hope in the caring relationship requires the nurse to see the possibilities of every moment with the client. Caring sometimes takes courage; courage is seen when the nurse provides care to the abusive, angry, and hostile client. When care is provided under poor staffing conditions, the nurse demonstrates courage. Courage is seen when a nurse questions the appropriateness of care. Caring is an integral aspect of patient care and is understood by patients and families in different ways (Mayeroff, 1971).

COMPETENCY FOR EVALUATING CARING PRACTICES

Sister M. Simone Roach (1992) describes the five "C's" of caring. They are: compassion, competence, confidence, conscience, and commitment. These five aspects of caring can be used to evaluate the concept of caring in a critical care nurse. Compassion is a quality of presence that allows the nurse to participate in the experience of the patient. Competence is a "state of having knowledge, judgment, and skills. It is the energy, experience, and motivation required responding adequately to the demands of one's professional responsibilities" (Roach, 1992, 61). Anticipating hazards and promoting safety, care, and comfort throughout transitions along the health care continuum is competence (AACN, 2003b). Confidence is a quality that must be present to ensure a trusting relationship with the patient and family. Nurses should put forth an aura of confidence in the delivery of care for patients and families to trust. Conscience is a moral awareness of being of service to others. Nurses should respond in an intentional, deliberate, meaningful manner. This way of being in the world while at the bedside is a display of consciousness. Lastly, commitment is characterized by a valued obligation to meet the needs of patients in a deliberate course of action (Hoover, 2002).

DEFINITION

Caring practices are the constellation of nursing activities that are responsive to the uniqueness of the patient and family needs. Creating a compassionate and therapeutic environment for promoting comfort and preventing suffering is the purpose of caring practices (AACN, 2002).

CASE STUDY

LB was a 77-year-old female who was admitted to the ICU after having gone to the emergency room with nausea and vomiting. During her time in the emergency department, she became nauseated and went into complete heart block, resulting in a cardiac arrest. The patient was resuscitated and brought to the ICU. On arrival to the ICU, she received an IV of normal saline at 100 cc/hr, oxygen at 2 liters nasal cannula, and was on the monitor in normal sinus rhythm. She was admitted with an uneventful history except for hypertension. During the assessment, her daughter and son remained present. The patient was asked if she had ever fallen at home; her answer was occasionally. The daughter stated that her mother was unsteady on her feet and had decreased strength over the past several months. The patient denied losing consciousness during her falls.

After the complete history was obtained, the daughter stated that hearing all of her mother's answers to the nurses' questions had been most informative and that she had learned a lot about her mother. After 6 hours of being in normal sinus rhythm, the patient developed second-degree block with a decreased blood pressure running systolically in the 80s. An external pacemaker was applied at a rate of 70 and an MA of 50. The patient complained of back pain from the external pacer electrode. The doctor was notified of the patient being symptomatic, and an order was received to set up for a transvenous temporary pacemaker. The family was notified and the patient was alert and oriented and signed the consent for the transvenous pacer. The transvenous pacer was placed femorally under fluoroscopy. The patient remained hemodynamically unstable for the next 4 hours requiring dopamine and intubation, and remained 100 percent paced. The family was allowed to remain at her bedside until the patient went into pulseless electrical activity (PEA).

At this point a code was called, and attempts at resuscitation were futile. The family was notified of their mother's death in a caring and supportive way. Information was provided as to the lengths taken to save her life and the disappointment that the team felt in being unsuccessful. The family had bonded with the nurse during the process of providing care to this patient, primarily because of the level of respect that had been afforded them, the continued updates provided to them throughout the patient's time in the critical care unit, and by the nurse being authentically present to the patient and family.

APPLICATION OF THE CASE STUDY TO THE SYNERGY MODEL

A Level 1 nurse focuses on the basic needs of the patient without anticipating future needs. Care is based upon standards and protocols. The nurse maintains a safe environment with a focus on improving disease specific outcomes. Death is considered a potential outcome. At Level 3, the nurse responds to subtle patient changes in a compassionate manner. Caring practices are tailored to the individual needs of the patient and family. The nurse provides small incidental acts of kindness during the course of care. Death is an acceptable outcome and supportive measures are designed to ensure a peaceful death. A Level 5 nurse has developed a heightened awareness that allows one to interpret the needs of patient and family. The nurse is capable of being fully engaged with the patient, family, and community in the design of care. Intuitiveness is utilized to sense the needs of the patient and family. The Level 5 nurse orchestrates the processes that ensure comfort and promote safety (AACN, 2002).

In this case, the nurse was working at a Level 5, primarily exhibited as an individual totally engaged in seeing the patient as a person and respecting the family in the process of providing care. The nurse ensured adequate communication with the family and extended their service as an intentional caring consciousness. The nurse promoted dignity in the care provided to the patient and family (AACN, 2003a).

REFERENCES

AACN. (2002). *Competency Level Descriptors for Nurse Characteristics*. Aliso Viejo, CA: AACN Certification Corporation.

AACN. (2003a). *CCRN Certification Blueprint for Study*. Aliso Viejo, CA: American Association of Critical Care Nurses.

AACN. (2003b). *Survey of Critical Care Nursing Practice*. Aliso Viejo, CA: American Association of Critical Care Nurses.

Blattner, B. (1981). Caring. In *Holistic Nursing,* B. Blattner (ed.). Englewood Cliffs, NJ: Prentice-Hall, Inc.

Burfitt, S. N., Greiner, D. S., Miers, L. J., Kinney, M. R., and Branyon, M. E. (1993). Professional Nurse Caring as Perceived by Critically Ill Patients: A Phenomenological Study. *American Journal of Critical Care* 2(6): 489–499.

Hoover, J. (2002). The Personal and Professional Impact of Undertaking an Educational Module on Human Caring. *Journal of Advanced Nursing* 37(1): 79–86.

Mayeroff, M. (1971). *On Caring*. New York: Barnes & Noble Books.

Patterson, G., and Zderad, L. T. (1976). *Humanistic Nursing*. New York: John Wiley & Sons, Inc.

Roach, M. S. (1992). *The Human Act of Caring: A Blueprint for the Health Professions,* rev. ed. Ottawa, Canada: Canadian Hospital Association Press.

Watson, J. (2001). Jean Watson Theory of Human Caring. In *Nursing Theories and Nursing Practice,* M. Parker (ed.). Philadelphia, PA: F. A. Davis, pp. 343–354.

CHAPTER 13

COLLABORATION

Sonya R. Hardin, PhD, RN, CCRN, APRN

Pharmaeg

INTRODUCTION

Throughout history, progress and even the survival of people have often depended on collaboration. When environmental conditions, competition, or other circumstances have made life more difficult or resources scarce, great civilizations and movements have been developed by people uniting for a common purpose. Collaboration enhances the capacity of a group and increases the potential for success. In this chapter, the concept of collaboration is presented followed by strategies for improving communication skills at the bedside. Strategies for developing nursing as a collaborative practice and evaluating collaboration as a competency are discussed. A case study is presented that demonstrates the utilization of collaboration to care for a complex critically ill client.

In a health care environment where resources are decreasing while demands are increasing, collaboration has become even more essential. Ensuring a safe passage for clients in health care facilities often requires extensive collaboration. Achieving optimal outcomes for clients evolves through the use of discovery, building, enhancing, and expanding existing strengths, assets, and resources of the patient and family. The presence or absence of collaborative relationships impacts patient care. Clients expect that their health care providers communicate and collaborate. Collaboration depends upon the establishment of collegial relationships (Hanson et al., 2000).

A key to collaboration is the communication that must exist between the patient, family, and health care team members as well as among members of the health care team. Communication skills include the sharing and collecting of information. Decisions should be shared and owned by all stakeholders. Finding the solution to difficult and complex client issues is best accomplished through collaboration.

COMMUNICATION SKILLS

Individuals that have a successful collaboration must have mutual respect, understanding, and trust for each other. Mutual respect for each person's knowledge and competence for the provision of quality care are essential to collaborative relationships (Scott et al., 1999). The existence of trust in a collaborative relationship ensures that decision making is shared, communication is not hampered, and coordination of care is well planned (Norsen et al., 1995). An open and frequent communication style among all individuals should be encouraged. During the communication process, do not interrupt. Allow the other person to complete their thought process to facilitate respectfulness. If you are an individual who tends to interrupt others, develop individualized methods to remind yourself to keep quiet. Methods that can be employed to remind yourself to stay quiet until the other person has finished talking include crossing your legs or holding both hands together until the other person has finished. Keep an open mind as the other person is speaking to increase communication (Almost & Laschinger, 2002). If you jump to conclusions or think a solution is the wrong approach before hearing the other person's completed proposal, collaboration can be impeded.

During an emotionally charged conversation, think through comments and carefully select words that will not be perceived negatively. Listening is a key skill in collaboration. Listen without planning on a response. Good listening often means asking good questions and clearing the mind of distractions. Barriers to listening often occur when an individual filters what is said, judges, daydreams, changes the subject, has a need to be the one who is right, or exhibits stonewalling behavior. Feedback to others is best accomplished through paying close attention to the thoughts and perspectives of all individuals. While listening to another, stay focused on the main points being presented. Respect the other person's point of view, even if you disagree with the approach being suggested. Be aware of nonverbal signs and mannerisms. The majority of messages are delivered through nonverbal signs (Stichler, 1995).

Never respond to another person's anger, even if they lash out in what seems a personal manner. Another person's mood or response is more likely about fear or frustration than it is about you as an individual. Take a deep breath and count to 10. See their anger as a way of letting the other person vent before he or she is able to communicate what is really on their mind (Norsen et al., 1995).

A professional should respond to facts and not feelings. When responding to charged feelings, respond by stating, "I understand your frustration" instead of "Hey, I'm just doing my job" or "It's not my job" (which is sure to cause more irritation). Understand that individuals want to be heard more than they care about whether you agree with them. You can show that you're listening by giving someone your complete attention and making statements such as: "Tell me more about your concern"; "What is it about _____ that concerns you?"; "I'm interested in what you've just said. Can you share a little bit about what led you to that belief?"; "What would have to happen for you to be more comfortable with _____?"

Remember also that what someone says and what you hear can be amazingly different! Our personal filters, assumptions, judgments, and beliefs can distort what you hear. Repeat back or summarize to ensure that you understand; re-state what you think you heard and ask, "Have I understood you correctly?" If you find yourself responding emotionally to what someone said, say so and ask for more information: "I may not be understanding you correctly, and I find my-self taking what you said personally. What I thought you just said is ____; is that what you meant?"

Do not offer advice unless asked. This can be difficult, particularly if you have experience that might benefit another person. A person can usually get a more positive response when respectful expressions are utilized, such as "One poten-tial option is . . ." or "One thing that helped me in a similar situation was ____. I'd be happy to share more about my experience if you think it'd be helpful to you" instead of "You should do ____."

COLLABORATION IN NURSING

Health care facilities have formulated teams to provide care to complex clients or focused on high volume Diagnosis Related Groups. Typically a team is formed based on the expertise needed to provide problem solving for specific client prob-lems. Collaboration can take the form of requesting the services of a specialized team to solve a challenging case. However, collaboration can also take place through the interactions of dyads between nurse–physician, nurse–respiratory therapist, nurse–dietician, nurse–nurse, nurse–environmental services, nurse–clinical engineering, nurse–speech therapist, and so forth. Effective planning of care to meet the needs of critically ill patients with complex, multisystem prob-lems and their families requires a multidisciplinary approach in order to attain timely and optimal outcomes (Relf and Kaplow, in press).

Many levels of collaboration can exist within an organization. Individuals can be coached and mentored in the skills needed to be collaborative. Learning the art of communication with the ability to present with openness to other thoughts and impressions of a case is part of the culture that can be established in an organiza-tion. New nurses often participate in team meetings. During these team meetings, new nurses share facts of the case and are seeking clarification and an enhanced understanding of the best practice in the delivery of services to the client. Nurses who have been working in their setting for a consistent period of time are often at a level to initiate and participate in team meetings or to initiate discussion with individuals who have the expertise needed to solve client problems. At this level, an experienced nurse has the skills to identify that the client's problems require a level of specialized expertise or a group that needs to have a shared vision for the outcomes of the client. An advanced practice nurse will seek opportunities to teach, coach, and mentor other nurses during the problem-solving process or team meeting. Through prior experiences, the advanced practice nurses have devel-oped the knowledge required to address complex client situations. Collaboration with other disciplines is often arranged by the advanced practice nurse through her prior experience and knowledge. At this level, the nurse is usually responsi-ble for the selection of team members who will best facilitate patient outcomes. The collaboration skills needed have evolved over the course of several years and include experience in working with others in a respectful and mutual goal-setting culture. Effectively utilizing the available resources to enhance patient care is the goal of an advanced practice nurse. Empirical data exist supporting the value of a collaborative working environment between nurses and physicians in the ICU setting. A collaborative relationship has been linked to higher job satisfaction and retention of nurses, higher level of patient satisfaction, and lower-than-expected mortality rates and patient length of stay (Relf and Kaplow, in press).

COMPETENCY FOR EVALUATING COLLABORATION

Numerous articles have been published that suggest a variety of skills that should exist to have competency in collaboration (NJPC, 1979; Spross, 1989; Evans, 1994; Stichler, 1995). Authors agree that many characteristics are essential for collaboration. Essential characteristics found in the literature include nurse autonomy, mutual trust and respect, an understanding and acceptance of another's discipline (NJPC, 1979), positive self-image, equivalent professional maturity arising from education and experience, recognition that the partners are not substitutes for each other (Spross, 1989), a willingness to negotiate, communication, goal sharing, task interdependence, a common purpose, and a sense of humor (Evans, 1994).

Those individuals who have developed the essential characteristics of collaboration can be viewed as experts in collaboration. Collaboration is a development process that occurs and matures over time. The fact that collaborative relationships are time dependent can explain why collaborative relationships can be less effective in organizations that have a high nurse turnover rate or a high usage of temporary staff.

Team participation requires the nurse to facilitate active involvement and contribute to team meetings. Participating fully as a team member is a competency for collaboration (AACN, 2003b).

DEFINITION

Collaboration is defined as working with others, including physicians, families, and health care providers in a way that promotes and encourages each person's contributions toward achieving optimal realistic patient goals (AACN, 2002). Individuals working in intra- and interdisciplinary teams provide an environment for an interactive process for problem solving. All members of a team share responsibility for ensuring holistic and safe care for clients (AACN, 2003a).

CASE STUDY

The following case study demonstrates the nurse characteristic of collaboration and actually occurred in a 16-bed critical care unit. The names have been changed to protect the confidentiality of the patient.

K was an 18-year-old Caucasian female who was admitted through the emergency department with a diagnosis of hypokalemia. Her potassium level on admission was 1.9. She was 5-foot, 8-inches tall and weighed 84 pounds. She had straight, shoulder-length hair, and her nails were bitten down to the skin. She appeared weak and unconcerned about her condition. When she was hooked up to the monitor, her EKG showed multifocal PVCs with a heart rate of 54. She had a peripheral IV of D5½NS infusing at 100 cc/hour. Her temperature registered 94 degrees Fahrenheit with the tympanic thermometer. On admission, she admitted to exercising daily and eating only low-fat foods. She stated that she ate a lot of pickles because they were filling and low calorie. Her eating pattern included occasional binging. She no longer had a menstrual cycle, about which she stated, "it makes life easier." On admission, she complained of being cold and warm blankets were provided for her. K said that she had always been "fat." The kids at school use to make fun of her and then the year following elementary school, she found the strength to start exercising and eating healthy. She stated that at age 11 she was a size 14 and was embarrassed to go shopping for clothes. Over the summer before starting 7th grade, she was down to a size 12, and by the middle of the fall semester was wearing a size 10. She continued to exercise and eat only low-fat foods. At times she would be hungry, but by Christmas of her 7th grade, she no longer felt hunger. "Actually, I was never hungry again and lost taste for all food." From that point on, it was a spiral down to a size 1. When she started high school, her parents decided that she needed to go to a therapist. K stated that the therapist told her parents that there was nothing psychologically wrong with her. She continued to see different therapists at her parents' insistence. Then one day, a therapist told her parents that she had anorexia and that it was brought on by obsessive compulsive disorder. K states, "I don't believe that I am anorexic or compulsive."

Physician orders state that someone is to stay in the room with her during meals and 1 hour afterwards to ensure that she eats and does not throw up. Orders included potassium levels every 6 hours with K+ runners of 10 Meq times 10 doses. In his progress notes, the physician had discussed inserting a feeding tube if improvement was not seen. The nurses providing care to the patient resented having to spend so much time with someone who they stated, "clearly wants to die, so why are we doing all of this?" The staff felt stretched to cover K's needs as well as take care of the rest of their assignments. K would move the food around on her plate and take only a few small bites in an hour, and then insist on going to the bathroom alone. Orders had been written that forbade her from being alone in the bathroom. Some nurses were uncomfortable with the instructions and questioned whether or not patient rights played into this case.

After 3 days, the physician decided that the patient needed a feeding tube and wanted it placed against the patient's will. The physician suggested that sedation be given to insert the tube. J, a registered nurse with 20 years of critical care experience, was caring for K on the day this order was written. She consulted the director of critical care and voiced her concern that this was not an appropriate order. The director suggested that she contact the psychiatric clinical nurse specialist (CNS) to get help on this case.

The psychiatric CNS scheduled an afternoon meeting with K. After talking to the patient, the CNS stated that the patient was competent and capable of making an informed decision about her care. The CNS spoke to the primary nurse and all the nurses in the unit regarding the diagnosis of anorexia. The CNS stated that anorexia nervosa is a life-threatening eating disorder that includes an intense fear of gaining weight, a distorted body image, and amenorrhea. Sometimes people starve and binge-purge, depending on the extent of weight loss. Conservative estimates suggest that $\frac{1}{2}$ to 1 percent of females in the United States develop anorexia (MacDonald, 2002).

The CNS initiated discussions with the physician, who continued to support his intervention of a feeding tube. The CNS decided to call the ethics committee together to get a multidisciplinary review of the case before any physician orders were carried out. During the evening hours, the ethics committee, the CNS, the physician, and the primary nurse met to discuss the case with the patient. At the completion of this meeting, a consensus was not reached. The psychiatric CNS scheduled a second meeting the following day after all participants had a chance to reflect on the patient's wishes. The next morning, the psychiatric CNS convened the meeting. Through the use of strong communication skills, she began the meeting by stating that all members were brought together to offer a perspective from their discipline that would help in solving the problem. She got all members to agree that the purpose and goal of the group was to develop a plan of care for K. She said that she respected each person's opinion and wanted to be clear that ultimately the patient had the final say in her treatment. The meeting lasted for 2 hours with discussion on the ethics of force feeding the patient, the rights of the client to choose or not choose interventions, and the best treatment options for the client. At the conclusion of the meeting, the decision was made that all health care professionals believed that K did not see her anorexia as a problem. The goal was to get her physiologically stable through electrolyte administration and that on admission to the emergency room, the goal would be medical stabilization of electrolytes and that no forced feedings would occur. The health care professionals were honest with K in stating that each of them felt that her health would continue to worsen unless she changed her eating behavior. They were extremely clear in stating that they believed that she would not live long. K continued to state that she was fine and basically that this admission was "just a little bump in the road." When the meeting ended, the CNS had a debriefing with members of the health care team. They discussed their feelings of helplessness in observing a person who was starving. The CNS continued to reinforce the rights of the patient to choose in her disease process and that they, as providers, had to support the decision of the client even if the client's choice was not consistent with theirs.

APPLICATION OF THE CASE STUDY TO THE SYNERGY MODEL

Anorexia nervosa is a multidimensional psychiatric disorder characterized by weight loss and distorted body image that is typically accompanied by denial. More than 90 percent of cases occur in females and anorexia nervosa is thought to have a long-term mortality rate of over 10 percent with most dying from starvation, suicide, or electrolyte imbalance (MacDonald, 2002). Little attention has been given to the ethical aspects of dealing with treatment resistance in an intensive care setting. These patients may resist treatment by; refusing to eat, using a naso-gastric tube for feedings, the covert use of laxatives and exercise. Treatment resistance often leads health care professionals to a quandary as to the best approach to take in the delivery of care. The patient's autonomy must be respected while designing a plan of care that both the practitioners and the patient can accept. Often the conflict arises when the treatment is perceived negatively by the patient. The use of collaboration in establishing a compromise among providers and patient is essential.

The CNS is a person capable of speaking both the languages of nursing and medicine. An understanding of each subculture assists the CNS in clinical problem solving. An advanced practice nurse should be an expert in collaboration and be able to role model the characteristics inherent in the role of collaborator. The CNS was practicing in an autonomous manner and utilizing conflict resolution skills in the negotiation of client care. The meetings were handled in a professional manner with the goal clearly stated and the establishment of mutual respect for all members.

REFERENCES

AACN. (2002). *Competency Level Descriptors for Nurse Characteristics*. Aliso Viejo, CA: AACN Certification Corporation.

AACN. (2003a). *CCRN Certification Blue Print for Study*. Aliso Viejo, CA: American Association of Critical Care Nurses.

AACN. (2003b). *Survey of Critical Care Nursing Practice*. Aliso Viejo, CA: American Association of Critical Care Nurses.

Almost, J., and Laschinger, H. K. (2002). Workplace Empowerment, Collaborative Work Relationships, and Job Strain in Nurse Practitioners. *Journal of the American Academy of Nurse Practitioners* 14(9): 408–420.

Evans, J. A. (1994). The Role of the Nurse Manager in Creating an Environment for Collaborative Practice. *Holistic Nursing Practice* 8(3): 23–31.

Hanson, C. M., Spross, J., and Carr, D. B. (2000). Collaboration. In *Advanced Nursing Practice: An Integrative Approach*, 2nd ed., A. B. Hamric, J. A. Spross, and C. M. Hanson (eds.). Philadelphia: W. B. Saunders Company, pp. 315–347.

MacDonald, C. (2002). Treatment Resistance in Anorexia Nervosa and the Pervasiveness of Ethics in Clinical Decision Making. *Canadian Journal of Psychiatry* 47: 267–270.

NJPCP. (1979). *Brief Description of a Demonstration Project to Establish Collaborative or Joint Practice in Hospitals*. Chicago: National Joint Practice Commission, pp. 2–6.

Norsen, L., Opladen, J., and Quinn, J. (1995). Practice Model: Collaborative Practice. *Critical Care Nursing Clinics of North America* 7(1): 43–52.

Relf, M., and Kaplow, R. (in press). Critical Care Nursing Practice: An Integration of Caring, Competence, and Commitment to Excellence. In *Critical Care Nursing: A Holistic Approach*, P. G. Morton, D. Fontaine, C. M. Hudak, and B. M. Gallo, (eds.). Philadelphia: Lippincott, Williams & Wilkins.

Scott, J. G., Sochalski, J., and Aiken, L. (1999). Review of Magnet Hospital Research: Findings and Implications for Professional Nursing Practice. *Journal of Nursing Administration* 29(1): 9–19.

Spross, J. A. (1989). The CNS as Collaborator. In A. B. Hamric and J. A. Spross, eds. *The Clinical Nurse Specialist in Theory and Practice,* 2nd ed. Philadelphia: W. B. Saunders Company, pp. 205–226.

Stichler, J. K. (1995). Professional Interdependence: The Art of Collaboration. *Advanced Practice Nursing Quarterly* 1(1): 53–61.

CHAPTER 14

SYSTEMS THINKING

Sonya R. Hardin, PhD, RN, CCRN, APRN

INTRODUCTION

Critical care nurses are confronted daily with situations that require them to solve patient problems. Often these problems are complex and can be at the individual, unit, division, organization, or community level. To effectively solve problems, nurses must be able to identify the real causes and view the problem holistically in relationship to all aspects of the system. Without a holistic view of the organization, nurses may be tempted to focus only on the behaviors and events associated with the problems, rather than on the system structures that underlie the problem in the first place. Systems thinking is a way of viewing the world by looking at the structures, patterns, and events of an issue, rather just the issue itself. There are certain principles that guide one to look through a holistic lens. These principles emerge over time as one's level of expertise increases. This chapter will discuss systems thinking and the implications for systems thinking in the AACN Synergy Model.

Initially, systems thinking was introduced in 1958 by MIT professor Jay Forrester. Forrester proposed a different way to the solution of a problem by shifting to a holistical analysis instead of through separating the problem into individual pieces (traditional method). Hence, systems thinking is a method of focusing on how a problem interacts with other aspects of the system. In this way, large numbers of interactions should be analyzed for each problem. The character of systems thinking makes it extremely effective on the most difficult types of problems to solve: those involving complex issues, those that depend a great deal on the past or on the actions of others, and those stemming from ineffective coordination among those involved (Aronson, 1996). Systems thinking should be utilized to solve complex problems that involve many participants, recurring problems or those that have been made worse by past attempts to fix, and problems whose solutions are not obvious.

In 1990, Peter Senge published *The Fifth Discipline*, a book suggesting that organizations shift their thinking to a learning organization if they were to be profitable. However, this book left executives wanting to implement systems thinking with their organizations, yet unsure about the procedures to utilize in delivery of these ideas. In 1994, Senge and colleagues published *The Fifth Discipline Fieldbook,* which gives more explicit direction on the strategies for enhancing the performance of an organization. A criticism of systems thinking is that many approaches and tools are esoteric and difficult for employees to apply.

Senge (1990) defines the essence of systems thinking as a shift of mind to (a) see interrelationships rather than linear cause-effect chains and (b) see processes of change rather than moments in time. Problem analysis should focus on the dynamic complexity of the situation and improving organizational work flow should emerge through the use of teams. Team effectiveness is seen when a team's output exceeds the sum of individual outputs (Moore New Products, 1995). French and Bell (1995) consider teams to be the "fundamental units of organization" and the "key leverage points for improving the functioning of the organization" (p. 171). Characteristics that make a team successful include a clear, elevating goal; a results-driven structure; competent team players; unified commitment; a collaborative climate; standards of excellence; external support and recognition; and principled leadership (French and Bell, 1995; Larson and LaFasto, 1989). In order for a team to be effective, Senge (1990) discusses the importance of team learning. In order for team learning to occur, all members must suspend their assumptions, regard each other as colleagues, and select a facilitator. Hierarchy is antithetical to dialogue and can stifle learning. Often, the centralization and use of hierarchy as the primary avenue for problem solving is less effective than allowing a team to strategize solutions.

Systems thinking can impact team performance. Senge and colleagues (1994) discuss four levels of a system integrated within a team. The most observable level within the structure of teams is the qualities of unspoken actions exhibited by members. A second level within a team is purpose. Each member of a team may be driven by a different purpose or goal. These purposes can reveal a personal need, a need for meaning, or a need for power. Authority and boundaries, and one's ego, will need to be explored if a team is going to be successful in solving a problem. Once a team forms to improve a process or to solve a problem, change is inevitable. The emphasis of the change should be focused on improving the entire organization. Senge (1990) identifies a number of concepts that are important to understand given systems thinking: causal loops, archetypes, and systems modeling.

Causal Loops

Causal loop is a structure used by systems thinkers to view the interrelationships of an organization. With a causal loop, a group looks at all the forces at work on the problem. Every variable impacting the problem should be listed as a cause or an effect that forms a circle surrounding the problem or situation being analyzed. Diagramming a loop may be complicated because of the many details associated with an event or problem. One of the problems observed in health care organizations is the lack of reflection in solving personnel, managerial, and financial problems. Because problems are not typically analyzed from a systems thinking perspective, problems continue to perpetuate.

Archetypes

Archetypes are universal symbols or models which other things are patterned after. These imprints or patterns are interconnected and can unfold unconsciously as a meaningful idea. Essentially, an archetype is a representation of the underlying structure of a process or event or object that influences behavior.

Systems Modeling

Systems modeling provides a framework for organizational change. Process mapping and simulation are often utilized to analyze processes within an organization. Process mapping will show the consequences when changes are made within an organization. It will explain both the external and internal boundaries and interdependencies associated with a problem. With simulation, one can observe behavior over time in a redesign scenario. Various software programs exist to educate executives in systems thinking. Before change is implemented, it is imperative that consequences are analyzed (Bierma, 2003).

A behavioral simulation game developed by MIT is the Beer Distribution Game, which requires players to choose an action based upon a situation. This game demonstrates that systems thinking controls the outcome regardless of who is at the helm. Players are shown how their decisions impacted the erratic results of the company. Even though this game takes half a day to play, valuable lessons are learned by management. The most important lesson experienced is how poor management practices can impact the whole system (Stumpf et al., 1994).

Lastly, Senge (1990) identifies six learning disabilities associated with the failure to think systematically. These learning disabilities operate on the individual, group, and organizational levels. The disabilities prevent individual learning and systems thinking, which ultimately contribute to dysfunctional systems. The first learning disability is "I am my position." The employees are so absorbed in being a nurse that they function as the role and not as human beings. People see their role in such a manner that only they have the ability to impact patient care.

"The enemy is out there" is a stance of blaming the organization for personal failure or problems. Nurses fall into this category when they start feeling like helpless victims of the organization. The nurse does not view her- or himself as capable of changing the system. "The illusion of taking charge" is often seen in the nurse who rises to the foreground during a crisis. This person has an opinion on every initiative and for an initiative to be successful, it must have their approval. This person treats the parts and does not consider the system. These individuals cannot see the forest for the tree standing in front of them. Their focus is narrow and on short-term outcomes. This is the quick-fix person who does not have a holistic perspective.

"The parable of the boiled frog" refers to the frog that jumps out of boiling water because it cannot adjust to a sudden change. However, when a frog is placed in cool water and the water temperature is gradually increased, the frog does not jump out of the water. The frog is unable to adjust to sudden changes in the environment, which is true of employees within organizations when sudden change occurs. Nurses must learn to adapt quickly to sudden change or they may jump out of the organization without warning.

"The delusion of learning from experience" sets individuals up for choosing solutions that may fail. Many of the problems seen today in health care are new and require new solutions. Repeating old solutions for new problems does not solve the issue.

The sixth learning disability, "the myth of the management team," is a group that comes together and reaches agreement on the surface but never has the courage to share deeply felt beliefs. Often, individuals go about their different ways and ignore group consensus because of deeply held beliefs about the decision.

DEFINITION

Systems thinking is a body of knowledge and tools that empowers the nurse to manage environmental and system resources for the patient or family and staff, within or across health care and nonhealth care systems (AACN, 2002). Based on the tenets of the AACN Synergy Model, a nurse at a Level 1 competency is often unclear on the steps to resolve a problem and therefore will utilize previously learned strategies or standardized processes. The worldview of the Level 1 nurse is within the narrow focus of the nursing unit. Nurses at this level see themselves as a key resource for the patient and family while working to meet the needs of the patient and family through the lens of their own personal experience. A Level 3 nurse has gained expertise over time in obtaining and utilizing resources within the health care system. Caring strategies are based upon the needs and strengths of the patient and family. The Level 3 nurse has the ability to recognize and react to the patients as they move through the health care system. The use of negotiation skills are utilized for practice-based decisions. Negotiation takes into consideration the needs of the patient and family and the resources available to provide best practices. Nurses who can recognize holistic interrelationships that exist within and across both health care and nonhealth care systems are at Level 5. At this level, a nurse utilizes a variety of resources, can anticipate the needs of the patient, and develops a variety of care strategies that are driven by the needs of the patient and family. A Level 5 nurse knows how to navigate through the system and use systems thinking on behalf of the client to ensure safe passage.

The nurse should develop, integrate, and apply a variety of strategies that are driven by the needs of patients and families. Utilizing proven strategies and developing creative strategies is a skill that ensures systems thinking competency. Recognition of holistic interrelationships that exist within and across the health care system is an example of systems thinking (AACN, 2003b).

An example that illustrates the difference between the systems thinking perspective and the perspective taken by traditional forms of analysis is the action taken to reduce vacancy rates in the staffing schedule. When a manager is faced with many shifts not being covered by the unit, the quickest fix at the moment might be to put all staff into mandatory overtime. According to this perspective, the more nurses are expected to work, the more likely shifts will need to be covered. The temptation is to say that eliminating the holes in the schedule will solve the problem; however, that often turns out to not be the case. The problem of staffing due to insufficient numbers does get better in the short term. Unfortunately, the long-term impact of mandatory scheduling can breed contempt and increase absenteeism, low morale, and burnout among staff. In other words, the action intended to solve the problem actually makes it worse because the unintended side effects change the system and end up creating other problems.

CASE STUDY

DZ was a 27-year-old male patient admitted to the telemetry unit diagnosed with rule out infective endocarditis. DZ was married with three children ages 2, 4, and 6. He was thin, emaciated, frail, and had a fever, swollen cervical nodes and a history of night sweats, myalgia, fatigue, and of lymphoma 2 years prior for which he received chemotherapy. On this admission, he admitted to his nurse that he had a history of intravenous drug use. Upon further questioning of lifestyle behaviors, a decision was made to test him for acquired immunodeficiency syndrome. He tested positive for HIV-1 antibody on enzyme-linked immunosorbent assay (ELISA), and the finding was confirmed by a Western blot test. Further results revealed that he was in the advanced stages of AIDS, with HIV-1 RNA levels exceeding 1 million copies per ml and low T-lymphocyte counts.

The challenges in this case were to 1) tell the patient of his HIV status, 2) discuss with the patient exposed contacts (i.e. wife and children) for contact tracing, 3) refer to an HIV-experienced General Practitioner (GP), and 4) notify the public health authorities. The patient was informed of his diagnosis and agreed to have the physician discuss the diagnosis with the wife. The wife was emotionally devastated requiring counseling. The wife and children where tested for HIV. The wife tested positive while all three children were negative. The wife required referral to an HIV-experienced GP and to a counselor. The hospital counselor met with the wife daily during her husband's week long in-patient visit. The wife agreed to take her husband home and to continue to live as a family unit. Due to DZ's debilitated state at discharge he required a case manager to work with several system issues. The patient had the following needs: 1) financial for drugs, 2) nutritional due to malnutrition, 3) child care for wife to continue working, 4) in-home medical care, 5) home-delivered meals, 6) education on recommendations to help patient avoid exposure to infections with opportunistic pathogens, and 7) end-of-life decisions (Mullahy, 1998). The case manager had to work with a number of different systems to acquire the resources that DZ and his wife needed. After one month of using home health resources a decision was made to bring in hospice. DZ died three months later in his home with his family at his bedside.

APPLICATION OF THE CASE STUDY TO THE SYNERGY MODEL

In approaching the problem from a systems thinking perspective, a long-term solution was to consider the needs of the patient and the resources in the community available to the patient and family. One must look at the big picture of how the daily life of this family will require as much normalcy as possible. Solving the problems related to financial, nutritional, child care, home care, and end-of-life decisions required the nurse to provide numerous interventions. Systems thinking has the power to help individuals create insights into problems that are complex, involve multiple individuals, and are at a level requiring more than one intervention.

Nurses at Level 1 will approach systems thinking by using resources readily available to meet the needs of the patient and family. They use protocols, policies, and guidelines to solve problems. Nursing care is provided based upon physiological needs of the patient without looking at the patient now and in the future. A Level 1 nurse will provide nursing care based on previously learned strategies or standardized processes that have previously been successful. For example, in this case a Level 1 nurse would follow a pathway for newly diagnosed HIV clients. This would have the nurse make standard referrals.

A Level 3 nurse will design strategies based on the needs, strengths and weaknesses of the patient and family. At this level, the nurse can recognize and utilize resources beyond self and see the importance of the transition process that patient and families will move through as they progress. A Level 3 nurse would recognize that the family would need child care given the debilitated state of the patient and that food preparation in the home would need to be obtained from an outside source.

A Level 5 nurse has the ability to develop, integrate, and apply various alternative and individualized strategies for solving patient problems (AACN, 2002). A global view allows for an ability to negotiate and navigate the patient through the system. At Level 5, the nurse is capable of working in the role of case manager. In this role, a global perspective is required to view the client holistically and to identify all needs given the many facets of the patient's life.

Systems thinking is a competency that emerges when the nurse has obtained the basic skills of caring for the physiological needs of the patient. Effective patient problem solving often requires the nurse to be able to understand how the system contributes to the problem. Without a clear understanding of the "big picture" of a system, nurses will focus on individual behaviors associated with the problem (AACN, 2003a).

REFERENCES

AACN. (2002). *Competency Level Descriptors for Nurse Characteristics*. Aliso Viejo, CA: AACN Certification Corporation.

AACN. (2003a). *CCRN Certification Blueprint for Study*. Aliso Viejo, CA: American Association of Critical Care Nurses.

AACN. (2003b). *Survey of Critical Care Nursing Practice*. Aliso Viejo, CA: American Association of Critical Care Nurses.

Aronson, D. (1996). Introduction to Systems Thinking. *Thinking Page.* Available at: www.thinking.net. Accessed April 26, 2004.

Bierema, I. L. (2003). Systems Thinking: A New Lens for Older Problems. *Journal of Continuing Education in the Health Professions* 23(2): S27–S33.

Forrester, J. W. (1958). Industrial Dynamics—A Major Breakthrough for Decision Makers. *Harvard Business Review* 36(4): 37–66.

French, W. L., and Bell, C. H. (1995). *Organization Development: Behavioral Science Interventions for Organization Improvement*, 5th ed. Englewood, NJ: Prentice-Hall, Inc.

Larson, C. E., and LaFasto, F. M. J. (1989). *Teamwork: What Must Go Right/ What Can Go Wrong.* Newberry Park, CA: Sage.

Moore New Products. (1995). *Facilities* 13(5): 15–16.

Mullahy, C. M. (1998). *The Case Manager's Handbook,* 2nd ed. Gaithersburg, MD: An Aspen Publication.

Senge, P. (1990). *The Fifth Discipline: The Art and Practice of the Learning Organization.* New York: Currency/DoubleDay.

Senge, P., Kleiner, A., Roberts, C., Ross, R., and Smith, B. (1994). *The Fifth Discipline Fieldbook.* New York: DoubleDay.

Stumpf, S. A., Watson, M. A., and Rustogi, H. (1994). Leadership in a Global Village: Creating Practice Fields to Develop Learning Organizations. *Journal of Management Development* 13(8): 16–25.

CHAPTER 15

RESPONSE TO DIVERSITY

Sonya R. Hardin, PhD, RN, CCRN, APRN

INTRODUCTION

The United States is experiencing a shift in demographic trends that reflect an increase in the diversity of the population. African Americans, American Indians, Alaska Natives, Asian Americans, Pacific Islanders, and Hispanic Americans accounted for 30 percent of the population in 2000 (U.S. Department of Health and Human Services, 2001a).

Nurses function in an environment that mirrors the diversity of the larger society. The diversity of patients is varied and related to gender, age, socioeconomic status, education, physical and mental abilities, regional locations, sexual lifestyle, and racial and ethnic background. In addition, the wave of new immigrants presents numerous issues (Dennis and Small, 2003; Suzuki et al., 2001). An understanding of the issues that arise due to cultural differences is necessary to ensure sensitivity to the needs of individuals, families, and groups who represent diverse cultural populations within our society. Health care providers must respect cultural beliefs and practices, including religious beliefs, dietary needs, personal care needs, daily routines, communication needs, and cultural safety needs (Dennis and Small, 2003).

RESPONSE TO DIVERSITY SKILLS

One of the first skills required in providing culture-specific care is personal awareness of one's own cultural assumptions and acknowledgment that hospitals and biomedicine are themselves cultures that impact patients and families. Nurses should assess the individuals' rationale for their ill health and identify patients' expectations. Open discussion of treatment options and supporting the client's wishes are crucial to culture-specific care.

Communication is essential in providing appropriate care. Nurses should consider body stance, proximity, gestures, language, listening style, gender differences, and eye contact. Communication difficulties should be approached with interpreters. When language interpretation is required, it may seem simple to utilize a family member. However, the use of a family member may illicit distorted information because of the individual's need for privacy (Narayanasamy, 2003).

Each nurse has the professional responsibility to continue his or her professional education and to strive toward cultural competence. Three highly utilized theoretical models for cultural assessment can be found in the literature: Leininger (1990), Giger and Davidhizar (1995), and Camphina-Bacote (1996). The Leininger model suggests that cultural content should consist of educational, economic, political, legal, kinship, religious, philosophical, and technical concerns. Giger and Davidhizar (1995) propose that nurses should understand communication, space, time, environmental control, biologic variations, and social organizations. The Camphina-Bocata (1996) model presents cultural competence as competencies in cultural awareness, cultural knowledge, and cultural skills. Each of these models could be utilized within critical care practice. The advantage of utilizing such a model is to frame the approach for culture-specific care.

Nurses bring two cultures to the bedside: (1) the nurse's personal culture and preferences and (2) the culture of the health care organization. Both of these cultures must be balanced with the culture of the patient and family. The ability to give optimal care requires that nurses know their own feelings, beliefs, and attitudes. Nurses must recognize how their attitudes and values impact conscious and unconscious clinical decisions.

Nurses should remember to keep the individual in the foreground and the culture in the background because it is ultimately the individual who should be considered as unique. Individuals should not be stereotyped. Different generations and individuals within the same family may have different values and beliefs. Some individuals will assimilate and assume the cultural values of society while others will maintain or blend values. Nurses should remember that not all people identify with their ethnic cultural background (American Academy of Nursing, 1995).

COMPETENCY FOR EVALUATING RESPONSE TO DIVERSITY

The Office of Minority Health in the U.S. Department of Health and Human Services (DHHS) has developed national standards for culturally and linguistically appropriate services (CLAS) in health care. Fourteen standards have been identified to promote culturally responsive organizations. These standards are organized around three themes: (1) culturally competent care, (2) language access services, and (3) organizational supports for cultural competence. Three standards are relevant to the theme of culturally competent care (DHHS, 2001b, pp. 5–7):

1. Health care organizations should ensure that patients or consumers receive from all staff members effective, understandable, and respectful care that is provided in a manner compatible with their cultural health beliefs and practices and preferred language.

2. Health care organizations should implement strategies to recruit, retain, and promote at all levels of the organization a diverse staff and leadership who are representative of the demographic characteristics of the service area.
3. Health care organizations should ensure that staff at all levels and across all disciplines receive ongoing education and training in culturally and linguistically appropriate service delivery.

Health care workers should be competent in understanding the differences in culture between themselves and the patient. Skills include the ability to work with interpreters, resolve conflicts between staff and patients, and understand cultural differences on health promotion, disease prevention, diagnosis, treatment, and supportive, rehabilitative, and end-of-life care (DHHS, 2001b).

The nurse should demonstrate competency in recognizing practices based upon diversity that have potentially negative outcomes for the patient. Incorporating the patient's and family's values with evidence-based practice is a creative approach to displaying competency of response to diversity (AACN, 2003b). Not only should the nurse be competent to respond to patient diversity but also to the diversity of the health care culture. Helping patients to understand the health care system culture and the practices within the health care system ensures that the nurse is meeting the needs of the patient (AACN, 2003b).

DEFINITION

Diversity is a concept that embraces not only ethnic groups and people of color but also other marginal or vulnerable people in society (Dennis and Small, 2003). Response to diversity is the ability of the nurse to recognize, appreciate, and incorporate differences into the provision of care (AACN, 2002). Differences are specifically related to individuality, cultural differences, spiritual beliefs, ethnicity, family configuration, lifestyle, socioeconomic status, values, and beliefs regarding health care (AACN, 2003a). Numerous writers have identified the significance of understanding and integrating culture-specific care into practice. Henley and Scott (1999) provide a guide for the cultural and spiritual needs of multiethnic patients. A sensitive approach to language differences is an important aspect of responding to diversity. Sherer (1993) states that language differences cause prolonged treatment, delay in treatment, and response in treatment. Polaschek (1998) and Narayanasamy (2002) propose the need for cultural safety within the health care system. Health care providers need to engage patients as partners in care where respect and rapport is enhanced through cultural negotiation and compromise. Health care providers must promote trust and therapeutic relationships that are vital for the design of culture-specific nursing interventions.

CASE STUDY

The following case study will demonstrate the nurse characteristic of a Level 1 response to diversity. A 35-year-old male from Mexico who speaks very little English comes to the emergency room with his supervisor from his job. While on the job site, he goes to his boss, points to his chest, and vomits. The boss tells the nurse that his employee is having chest pain. The nurse tells the physician that the patient is having chest pain. The physician orders a STAT EKG at a cost of $220, STAT CPK Isoenzymes costing $125, electrolytes costing $55, CBC costing $45, and a STAT portable chest X-ray at a cost of $120. All test results were negative. A family member arrives who can speak English and acts as an interpreter. The family member tells the nurse that the patient is not having chest pain, but stomach pain. The patient is then worked up as having a gastrointestinal problem. An ultrasound of the gallbladder finds that the patient needs a cholecystectomy. The lack of communication cost the patient an extra $445.

APPLICATION OF THE CASE STUDY TO THE SYNERGY MODEL

A Level 1 nurse is capable of assessing cultural diversity through a standardized questionnaire. Nurses will typically provide care based on their own belief system. Nurses at Level 1 are in the process of learning about the culture of the health care environment and the functions of the organization. In this example, the nurse was responsive to the needs of the patient but did not seek out interpreter services for working with this patient. Conclusions were drawn based upon prior experience of associating chest pain with a potential myocardial infarction.

At Level 3, a nurse actively inquires about cultural differences and considers the individuality of the patient in the plan of care. Differences are incorporated and specific interventions are considered. The nurse works to educate the patient and family about the health care system and how to safely navigate the system. At Level 3, the nurse would have sought an interpreter for the case presented. A Level 5 nurse responds to, anticipates, and integrates cultural differences to the patient and family plan of care. Differences are incorporated into the plan of care with the clear ability to negotiate with the patient and family the differing values between the health care system and the individual. The diverse needs of the patient are considered in all clinical decisions, with alternatives being presented for patient involvement (AACN, 2003a).

REFERENCES

AACN. (2002). *Competency Level Descriptors for Nurse Characteristics*. Aliso Viejo, CA: AACN Certification Corporation.

AACN. (2003a). *CCRN Certification Blue Print for Study*. Aliso Viejo, CA: American Association of Critical Care Nurses.

AACN. (2003b). *Survey of Critical Care Nursing Practice*. Aliso Viejo, CA: American Association of Critical Care Nurses.

American Academy of Nursing. (1995). *Promoting Cultural Competence*. Washington, DC: American Academy of Nursing.

Camphina-Bacote, J. (1996). The Challenge of Cultural Diversity for Nurse Educators. *The Journal of Continuing Education in Nursing* 27: 59–64.

Dennis, B. P., and Small, E. B., (2003). Incorporating Cultural Diversity in Nursing Care: An Action Plan. *The Association of Black Nursing Faculty Journal* 1: 17–25.

Geron, S. M. (2002). Cultural Competency: How Is It Measured? Does It Make a Difference? *Generations* Fall: 39–45.

Giger, J. N., and Davidhizar, R. E. (1995). *Transcultural Nursing: Assessment and Intervention*, 2nd ed. St Louis, MO: Mosby.

Henley, A., and Scott, J. (1999). *Culture, Religion and Patient Care in a Multiethnic Society*. London: Age Concern.

Leininger, M. (1990). Issues, Questions and Concerns Related to the Nursing Diagnosis Cultural Movement from a Transcultural Nursing Perspective. *Journal of Transcultural Nursing* 2(1): 23–32.

Narayanasamy, A. (2002). The ACCESS Model: A Transcultural Nursing Practice Framework. *British Journal of Nursing* 11(9): 643–650.

Narayanasamy, A. (2003). Transcultural Nursing: How Do Nurses Respond to Cultural Needs? *British Journal of Nursing* 12(3): 185–194.

Polaschek, N. R. (1998). Cultural Safety: A New Concept in Nursing People of Different Ethnicities. *Journal of Advanced Nursing* 27(3): 452–457.

Sherer, J. L. (1993). Crossing Cultures: Hospitals Begin Breaking Down the Barriers to Care. *Hospitals* 67(10): 29–31.

Suzuki, L. A., McRae, M. B., and Short, E. L. (2001). The Facets of Cultural Competence: Searching Outside the Box. *The Counseling Psychologist* 29(6): 842–849.

U.S. Department of Health and Human Services. (2001a). *Mental Health: Culture, Race, and Ethnicity—A Supplement to Mental Health: A Report of the Surgeon General*. Rockville, MD: Author.

U.S. Department of Health and Human Services. (2001b). *National Standards for Culturally and Linguistically Appropriate Services in Health Care*. Rockville, MD: Author.

CHAPTER 16

CLINICAL INQUIRY

Sonya R. Hardin, PhD, RN, CCRN, APRN

INTRODUCTION

Clinical inquiry is the systematic questioning or investigation of events or circumstances related to improving patient care. When nurses have a question they believe should be answered to improve patient outcomes, they can conduct nursing research, conduct literature reviews, or utilize research findings from the literature. Nurses can contribute to nursing research by (Leddy and Pepper, 1998, p. 144):

1. Using nursing research findings to guide nursing practice
2. Valuing a sense of inquiry about the phenomena of nursing
3. Participating in research projects as opportunity allows
4. Refining ability to collect, organize, categorize, and analyze data
5. Suggesting the nursing research questions that need to be addressed to improve practice

CLINICAL INQUIRY SKILLS

Clinical inquiry begins with a clinical problem that requires a solution. Nurses identify a question in order to find the best answer for meeting the needs of patients. Greenlaugh (1997) identifies four components to a clinical question:

1. The patient problem
2. A connection between the problem and intervention
3. An alternative intervention
4. The outcome for the patient

For example, "Is the supine position the best position for an accurate cardiac output to ensure patient comfort and consistent measurements?"

Sackett and colleagues (2000) report that the nurse's level of experience influences the types of questions proposed. Less experienced nurses often ask basic information questions that build to their basic knowledge. The more experienced nurse often asks questions that are outcome-based questions. This is the best approach to seek to solve a clinical problem.

Secondly, the nurse should be capable of conducting a critical analysis of the literature. In reviewing the literature, the nurse must discern whether the information is valid and if the results can be applied to practice. Understanding the applicability of the study findings to practice is a clinical inquiry skill.

Lastly, a clinical inquiry skill is the ability of the nurse to perform a systematic review of the literature. This skill requires the nurse to look at all the research and to pool the results in such a manner as to identify trends that support practice. This is a high-level skill in that the nurse must understand internal validity, external validity, and reliability (Sams and Ritzert, 2003).

COMPETENCY FOR EVALUATING CLINICAL INQUIRY

For the nurse to be competent in clinical inquiry, several behaviors should be demonstrated. First, the nurse should display knowledge-seeking behaviors such as being open to advice, appreciating life-long learning, and seeking knowledge to address clinical questions. Second, the nurse needs to be competent in identifying clinical problems and searching for evidence in the literature to validate or change practice. Lastly, the nurse should be competent in participating in the research process. Participation includes being part of a team, collecting data, evaluating outcomes of studies, and bringing about change in practice based upon evidence (AACN, 2003b).

DEFINITION

Clinical inquiry is the ongoing process of questioning and evaluating practice, providing informed practice, and innovating through research and experiential learning (AACN, 2003a). Nurses should be engaged in clinical knowledge development to promote the best patient outcomes (AACN, 2002). The most significant step in clinical inquiry is when the nurse identifies a question that must be answered to increase professional understanding of a patient care issue. Nurses are accountable for asking questions that reflect sensitivity to the needs of patients and the interaction of the environment, health, and patient characteristics. Clinical inquiry, as described, could also be associated with a national movement to establish evidence-based practice through conducting research that supports nursing practice. Evidenced-based practice is an approach to care that is grounded on a critical review of relevant data such as research findings, retrospective chart reviews, quality improvement and risk management data, infection control data, and benchmarking data. Such data should guide practice and not tradition, organizational culture, or ritualistic practices.

CASE STUDY

JW is an 85-year-old man admitted to the critical care unit after having suffered from a massive myocardial infarction. He is currently being monitored with an EKG reading of atrial fibrillation with a ventricular rate of 110. He is on a Cardizem® (Diltiazem) infusion at 20 mg/min. His blood pressure is being managed with Intropin® (Dopamine) at 20 mcg/kg/min sustaining a B/P of 80/62. Urinary output is minimal at barely 30 cc/hr. He is intubated with a number 8 endotracheal tube at the 22 cm mark at the lip and ventilated on FIO2 at .60, TV 700, SIMV 10, Peep 5, and pressure support of 15 cm H_2O. He has crackles three quarters of the way up posteriorly and has a Lasix® (Furosemide) drip infusing at 10 mg/hour. On admission to the critical care unit, a pulmonary artery catheter was inserted. His pressure readings are 48/25 with a wedge pressure of 28 mmHg and a cardiac output of 3.6 l/m.

Thermodilution is the method utilized in this unit for cardiac output. Cardiac output is a measurement frequently ordered in the critical care unit and is the product of heart rate and the stroke volume and reflects the amount of blood in liters ejected from the left ventricle each minute. The value of a cardiac output in clinical practice is that it determines organ perfusion and oxygen delivery to the tissues.

The nurse caring for JW questions whether a difference exists in the position of the patient during cardiac output measurements. The unit policy states that the patient must be flat for the cardiac output to be performed. The nurse has noticed that the patient is uncomfortable in a flat position. Through inquiry, the nurse is lead to first conduct a literature review to see if this question has been previously researched. The nurse finds that several studies have been conducted, but they are limited. Of the four studies that have been conducted, several reported a decrease in the cardiac output with an elevated head of bed (Kleven, 1984; Wilson et al., 1996; Driscoll et al., 1995) and one reported no change when the position was changed (Grose et al., 1981). The nurse did not find a study where the measurement of time with position change had been considered. The evidence was inconclusive. Therefore, a study was proposed that would evaluate the cardiac output at three different points in time (0 minutes, 5 minutes, and 10 minutes) after a position change was made. Position changes consisted of a head-of-bed angle of 0°, 30°, and 45°. The nurse found no significant difference in the cardiac index (cardiac output/BSA) values across the nine different measurement conditions (Giuliano et al., 2003). The nurse realized that the patient condition often necessitates an elevation in the head of the bed. Given the data from the study, the nurse proposed a policy change in the unit. Semifowlers positioning is the recommended position for intubated patients who have no contraindication for having their head of the bed elevated (Giuliano et al., 2003). Questioning practice can lead to changes in policy and practices for the nurse at the bedside.

APPLICATION OF THE CASE STUDY TO THE SYNERGY MODEL

The nurse at Level 1 follows standards and guidelines that have been established by regulatory agencies and health care organizations. Clinical changes are implemented by incorporating research-based practices. The nurse recognizes the need for further learning to improve patient care. A Level 1 nurse recognizes obvious changes in the patient situation and seeks help in identifying patient problems (AACN, 2002).

A Level 3 nurse will question the appropriateness of policies and guidelines. Current practice is questioned. Patient care is improved through the nurse seeking advice, resources, and/or information. The nurse begins to compare and contrast possible alternatives (AACN, 2002).

The nurse at Level 5 will improve, deviate from, or individualize standards and guidelines for particular patient situations or populations. Current practice is questioned given patient response, review of the literature, research, and education. Questions that arise in practice are researched to gain knowledge that will improve patient care (AACN, 2002).

In this case study, the nurse is functioning at a Level 5. Current practice is questioned and the nurse seeks to research the literature for evidence that the practice of conducting cardiac outputs in the supine position is the method of choice. The review of the literature led the nurse to believe that sufficient data had not been collected and evaluated. Therefore, the nurse conducted a study utilizing more variables and found no difference associated with the position of the patient during cardiac output. Based upon the findings of the study, the nurse proposed a change in the policy and in current practice.

REFERENCES

AACN. (2002). *Competency Level Descriptors for Nurse Characteristics*. Aliso Viejo, CA: AACN Certification Corporation.

AACN. (2003a). *CCRN Certification Blue Print for Study*. Aliso Viejo, CA: American Association of Critical Care Nurses.

AACN. (2003b). *Survey of Critical Care Nursing Practice*. Aliso Viejo, CA: American Association of Critical Care Nurses.

Driscoll, A., Shanahan, A., Crommy, L., Foong, S., and Gleeson, A. (1995). The Effect of Patient Position on the Reproducibility of Cardiac Output Measurements. *Heart & Lung: Journal of Acute & Critical Care* 24: 38–44.

Giuliano, K. K., Scott, S. S., Brown, V., and Olson, M. (2003). Backrest Angle and Cardiac Output Measurement in Critically Ill Patients. *Nursing Research* 52(4): 242–248.

Greenlaugh, T. (1997). *How to Read a Paper: The Basics of Evidence Based Medicine*. London: BMJ Publishers.

Grose, B., Woods, S., and Laurent, D. (1981). Effect of Backrest Position on Cardiac Output Measured by the Thermodilution Method in Acutely Ill Patients. *Heart & Lung: Journal of Acute & Critical Care* 6(6): 452–456.

Kleven, M. (1984). Effect of Backrest Position on Thermodilution Cardiac Output in Critically Ill Patients Receiving Mechanical Ventilation with Positive End-Expiratory Pressure. *Heart & Lung: Journal of Acute & Critical Care* 13(3): 303–304.

Leddy, S., and Pepper, J. M. (1998). *Conceptual Bases of Professional Nursing*, 4th ed. Philadelphia: Lippincott.

Sackett, D. L., Rosenberg, W., Haynes, R. B., and Richardson, W. S. (2000). Evidenced Based Medicine: What It Is and What It Isn't. *British Medical Journal* 312: 71–72.

Sams, L., and Ritzert, B. (2003). Evidence-Based Practice and Nursing Research. In *Nursing in Contemporary Society: Issues, Trends, and Transition to Practice,* L. Haynes, T. Boese, and B. Howard (eds.). Upper Saddle River, NJ: Prentice Hall.

Wilson, A. E., Bermingham-Mitchell, K., Wells, N., and Zachary, K. (1996). Effect of Backrest Position on Hemodynamic and Right Ventricular Measurements in Critically Ill Adults. *American Journal of Critical Care* 5(4): 264–270.

CHAPTER 17

FACILITATOR OF LEARNING

Sonya R. Hardin, PhD, RN, CCRN, APRN

INTRODUCTION

A learning culture is one where people are creative in all their relationships and experiences. Such a culture encourages nurses to seek out opportunities to learn and teach others. *Learning* is a change in behavior resulting from practice and experience. *Teaching* is a plan of action to bring about learning. Teaching and learning are not separate entities but are synergistic in nature and interactive. The teaching-learning process involves assessing the learning needs of the patient, encouraging the patient to set goals, implementing strategies to convey information, and then evaluating understanding of content. This chapter describes the nurse's role in facilitating the learning of patients and families.

THEORIES OF LEARNING

The stimulus-response learning theory began in the 1930s when B. F. Skinner (1938) pioneered operant conditioning. Operant conditioning involved positive and negative reinforcements, spaced irregularly to make behavior permanent. Operant conditioning was the basis for "programmed instruction." This style of learning provides individuals with small units or modules of learning with immediate feedback about correct responses (Bigge, 1971).

Cognitive-field theory of learning was proposed in the 1940s by Kurt Lewin (1948). This theory assumes that a person, at whatever the level of understanding, does the best that they know how for whatever is thought to be best. Intellectual processes are deeply affected by an individual's goals. Goals are central to the cognitive-field theory of learning (Bigge, 1971).

The humanistic learning theory, in which value is placed on self-assessment and growth of the learner, was largely proposed by Carl Rogers (1969). The learner is motivated when the content is viewed as useful. Learning is acquired through the act of doing. The values of the patient are paramount, and learning will not occur if the patient does not value the purpose of learning (Lefrancois, 1975).

Every teaching-learning situation that the nurse encounters will contain principles from these three theories. All three of these theories are utilized in a holistic teaching-learning process.

FACILITATOR OF LEARNING IN NURSING

The purpose of educating patients is to maximize their creative potential, to examine and critique relevant issues, and to support patients living in their own unique way. The teacher is a resource for the patient and enhances each patient's unique cultural background, values, and life experiences. Nurses should assess the patient's learning style. Learning styles can be visual, aural, verbal, physical, logical, social, or solitary. Visual learners prefer to use pictures, images, and special understanding. Aural learners prefer using sound and music. They will remember something better if it is presented in a rhythm. Verbal learners prefer using words, both spoken and written. These individuals would benefit from pamphlets or videos. Physical learners prefer doing, using their hands, and the sense of touch. Logical learners would like a logical presentation of ideas, use of patterns displaying relationships, and information grouped categorically. Social learners prefer learning in groups by sharing ideas and reflecting on the comments of others. The use of games is conducive to the learning style of a social learner. Solitary learners are introspective, need time to reflect, and prefer to work independently on learning information. Self-study guides are useful among the solitary learner (Bigge, 1971).

COMPETENCY FOR EVALUATING FACILITATOR OF LEARNING

Nurses need skills to help the patient access health information but they are also required to interpret informational meaning and to sort out relevant information that fits the patient's needs. Information should be provided to increase patient knowledge of their diagnosis, illness, treatment needs, and behaviors needed to promote health. Assessment skills are needed to identify learning needs, abilities, and readiness (Arnold, 2003). Clear discharge instructions for the education level of the patient should be inclusive and coordinated with the patient's primary caregiver. Nurses should be capable of providing coordinated learning activities and resources based upon client and family needs. The ability to integrate the health care team into the teaching plan of patients and families to ensure a comprehensive approach to unique health care situation is a teaching competency for nurses. Evaluation of the patient and family's readiness to learn is a competency for facilitating learning (AACN, 2003b).

Given today's health care environment, teaching goals need to be measurable, realistic, and achievable in the time frame allotted. Choosing the most appropriate teaching strategies is often an advanced skill in nursing. Adjusting teaching strategies to meet the needs of the patient requires a high level of experience

(Arnold, 2003). Many patients will need creative teaching strategies to ensure the understanding of skills required for self-management. Another competency in the facilitator of learning characteristic includes the ability to present material in an informal one-to-one relationship, formal structured group sessions, or in a family conference setting (London, 2001). Lastly, as health care moves into the community with a case mix of unstable critically ill home care needs, a nurse must be capable of teaching the client for the purpose of optimal functioning and improved self-care management (Conley and Burman, 1997).

DEFINITION

Facilitator of learning is defined by AACN as the ability to facilitate patient and family learning (AACN, 2003a). The nurse should be capable of recognizing patient and family needs for information (AACN, 2002). Standardized educational materials, patient-centered education materials, and creative strategies for teaching can be utilized to ensure clients have the information needed to improve outcomes.

Nurses should be able to conduct needs assessments prior to structured education. Advanced practice nurses display the skill of delivering formal and informal intra- and interdisciplinary education to improve patient outcomes. Promoting the value of lifelong learning and evidence-based practice in the system is a skill of facilitator of learning (AACN, 2003b).

CASE STUDY

Mr. J is a 64-year-old man admitted to the coronary care unit. He has a history of hypertension, diabetes, and high cholesterol. His admitting diagnosis is R/O MI (rule out myocardial infarction). The physician orders include daily EKG, CPK Isoenzymes, and Troponin levels every 8 hours times three, a cardiac diet, 1800 calorie ADA diet, saline lock, routine vital signs, oxygen at 2 liters by nasal cannula, ACCU checks AC and HS, Humulin insulin on a sliding scale, Capoten® (Captopril) 25 mg tid, Zocor® (Simvastatin) 10 mg every day, and NPH insulin® 35 units every morning. The nurse receives the first set of isoenyzmes back from the lab showing elevated CPK and elevated Troponin levels. The EKG findings support the diagnosis of an anterior lateral MI.

The nurse approaches the patient to discuss his medication regime at home. During the discussion, the patient discloses that he has not been taking the prescribed Zocor® because he can only afford to buy his insulin and blood pressure medicine. Initially the nurse was approached by the patient asking why he had a heart attack. The patient questioning the nurse for information prompts the nurse to assess the patient's readiness to learn and to uncover his current level of knowledge. The nurse talks with the patient about the impact of cholesterol on the development of plaque in the coronary arteries and the benefits of Zocor®. The patient states that no one had ever explained the relationship of Zocor® to the prevention of having a heart attack. Then he realizes that the Zocor® is just as important as his other medications. In talking to the patient, the nurse has learned that the patient valued his insulin and blood pressure medicine in the prevention of disease but did not understand the usefulness of a cholesterol-lowering agent. His lack of knowledge led him to make uninformed choices. His choices were based upon his knowledge of the need to control his glucose level and blood pressure. The relationship of cholesterol and cardiac disease had not been understood by the patient.

APPLICATION OF THE CASE STUDY TO THE SYNERGY MODEL

This nurse is working as a Level 3 nurse. The patient was assessed for readiness to learn and prior knowledge. Information was shared with the patient and the nurse verified that he understood through verbal instructions.

The nurse at Level 1 follows planned education specific for the patient's disease process. The patient and family education are seen as separate components of care. Education is provided without assessing the patient's readiness to learn or prior knowledge. At Level 1, the patient is not viewed holistically, but as a passive recipient of information. No involvement of the patient is integrated into the educational program (AACN, 2003a). A Level 3 nurse begins to recognize that different methods of teaching should be considered given the unique needs of the patient. The patient is incorporated into the plan by assessing the patient's perspective of his needs and level of understanding. The patient and nurse develop educational goals given the individualistic needs of care (AACN, 2003a). At Level 5, the nurse works with the patient and family to develop an educational plan based on an evaluation of the patient's understanding. The nurse collaborates with the patient, family, and other health care disciplines to ensure that all educational needs are met. Realistic patient-driven goals are established and the patient understands the consequences of his choices (AACN, 2003a).

REFERENCES

AACN. (2002). *Competency Level Descriptors for Nurse Characteristics*. Aliso Viejo, CA: AACN Certification Corporation.

AACN. (2003a). *CCRN Certification Blueprint for Study*. Aliso Viejo, CA: American Association of Critical Care Nurses.

AACN. (2003b). *Survey of Critical Care Nursing Practice*. Aliso Viejo, CA: American Association of Critical Care Nurses.

Arnold, E. (2003). Health Teaching in the Nurse-Client Relationship. In *Interpersonal Relationships: Professional Communication Skills for Nurses*, E. Arnold and K. U. Boggs (eds.). St. Louis, MO: Saunders, pp. 410–437.

Bigge, M. L. (1971). *Learning Theories for Teachers*. New York: Harper & Row.

Conley, V., and Burman, M. (1997). Informational Needs of Caregivers of Terminal Patients in a Rural State. *Home Health Care Nurse* 15(11): 808–817.

Lefrancois, G. R. (1975). *Psychology for Teaching*. Belmont, CA: Wadsworth Publishing Co.

Lewin, K. (1948). *Resolving Social Conflicts*. New York: Harper and Brothers.

London, F. (2001). Take the Frustration Out of Patient Education. *Home Healthcare Nurse* 19(3): 158–160.

Rogers, C. (1969). *Freedom to Learn: A View of What Education Might Become*. Columbus, OH: Charles Merrill.

Skinner, B. F. (1938). *The Behavior of Organizations: An Experimental Analysis*. Norwood, NJ: Prentice Hall.

SECTION IV

SAMPLE QUESTIONS
OF THE AACN SYNERGY MODEL

CHAPTER 18

THE ACUTELY AND CRITICALLY ILL ADULT PATIENT SAMPLE QUESTIONS

Michael W. Day, MSN, RN, CCRN

INTRODUCTION

The following questions have been developed to provide examples of questions that integrate the patient and nurse characteristics of the AACN Synergy Model. The scenarios and questions in this chapter focus on acutely and critically ill adult patients in a variety of patient care settings. Each question is followed by four choices; one answer is correct. An annotated key at the end of the questions provides the correct choice along with a rationale for why the other choices are not the best, based on the AACN Synergy Model.

SCENARIO 1

Following a motor vehicle crash, a patient has just been admitted to the Intensive Care Unit (ICU) with a right pneumothorax, fractured pelvis, and pulmonary contusions. The following three questions relate to this scenario.

1. Which of the following are the most appropriate initial tasks?
   a. Ensure adequate ventilation, monitor for hemodynamic instability.
   b. Locate the patient's family, contact the on-call physician for an evaluation.
   c. Ensure adequate ventilation, locate the patient's family.
   d. Monitor for hemodynamic instability, contact the on-call physician for an evaluation.

2. As the patient recovers from the injuries incurred and is transferred to an acute care unit (ACU), he becomes insistent about establishing who may or may not be allowed to visit. Which of the following interventions would be most appropriate?

    a. Tell the patient that visiting rules only allow family members.
    b. Discuss the patient's request with the chaplain.
    c. Discuss the patient's request with the parents.
    d. Allow the patient to determine who visits.

3. Two days after his transfer to the ACU, the patient is readmitted to the
    ICU for increasing dyspnea, tachypnea, and productive cough, on 3 liters
    of oxygen via nasal cannula. A chest X-ray reveals normal lung expan-
    sion with right lower lobe infiltrates. Blood gases reveal a respiratory aci-
    dosis. Which of the following interventions would be most appropriate?
    a. Contact the on-call anesthesia provider for an immediate intubation.
    b. Apply a 100 percent nonrebreather oxygen mask.
    c. Ask the respiratory therapist for nebulizer treatment.
    d. Administer the next antibiotic dose early.

SCENARIO 2

A patient is admitted to the coronary care unit (CCU) following a two-vessel
coronary artery bypass graft (CABG). Due to a history of bronchitis, the patient
fails three attempts at weaning over the past 2 days. The physician decides to wait
a couple of days before attempting to wean again. The following five questions
relate to this scenario.

4. Which of the following interventions will be most helpful in assisting the
    patient to be successful with the next weaning attempt?
    a. Stimulate the patient to remain alert.
    b. Establish a routine of rest and activity.
    c. Provide encouragement to the patient.
    d. Deliver sedation to allow maximal rest.

5. Before the next extubation attempt, the physician orders a nutrition con-
    sult. Which of the following routes would be the most effective and safest
    way to deliver nutrition to this patient?
    a. Parental nutrition via a peripherally inserted central catheter (PICC).
    b. Enteral nutrition via a naso-duodenal (ND) feeding tube.
    c. Parental nutrition via a central venous catheter (CVC).
    d. Enteral nutrition via a precutaneous entero-gastric (PEG) tube.

6. The patient in Scenario 2 is successfully weaned and extubated 8 days after
    surgery. Which of the following would be the most appropriate consult?
    a. Physical therapy for strengthing exercises.
    b. Occupational therapy for ADL assistance.
    c. Speech therapy for swallow evaluation.
    d. Dietitian for nutrition evaluation.

7. The patient is transferred to an ACU where recovery continues. In talk-
    ing with the patient's spouse, the nurse learns that they live on the second
    floor of an apartment building that has no elevator. In addition, despite

repeated explanations, the spouse expresses a lack of understanding of the wound care and precautions the patient will need to take for the next couple of weeks. Which of the following interventions would be most appropriate?

a. Ask the patient's grown son to move in for a short time to provide care.
b. Reinforce information about wound care and provide reassurance to the spouse.
c. Consult with the patient's insurance carrier for nursing home placement.
d. Contact case management or social work for a home nursing consult.

8. Upon discharge, the social workers arranged for a home health nurse to visit the patient three times a week. One week after returning to the apartment, the patient reports to the home health nurse that he has noticed a decrease in strength and is finding it more difficult to maneuver around the apartment. Which of the following would be the most appropriate intervention on the part of the home health nurse?

a. Assess the patient for signs and symptoms of heart failure.
b. Arrange for an ADL consult with an occupational therapist.
c. Contact the physician for a direct admit to the hospital.
d. Arrange for the patient's grown son to provide daily help.

SCENARIO 3

A Native American from a nearby rural reservation is admitted from the emergency department (ED) to the ACU with a diagnosis of hepatic encephalopathy. The patient has a 25-year history of recurrent alcoholism and was found "down" in his home by his only child, a grown daughter who also lives on the reservation. She was unable to arouse him and called 911. The patient was transferred to the hospital by an air medical ambulance. The air medical crew noted that he was unresponsive at the scene and during the flight, but that he had maintained a blood pressure of 146/72, with a heart rate of 110. An oral airway was inserted and the patient was placed on a 100 percent nonrebreather. The following four questions relate to this scenario.

9. Based on this scenario, which of the following actions would be the most appropriate?

a. Establish the patient's code status with the grown daughter.
b. Arrange for a transfer to the ICU.
c. Assess the patient's hemodynamic and respiratory status.
d. Contact the patient's physician for orders.

10. Upon physical assessment, the patient is found to be jaundiced, nonresponsive but stable. The patient's abdomen is significantly distended, with visible fluid waves. Abdominal X-rays reveal massive ascites and the physician determines that a peritoneal tap is necessary to relieve pres-

ure on the diaphragm. The patient's grown daughter has signed an authorization for the procedure, but voices concerns to the nurse regarding its necessity. Which of the following would be the nurse's most appropriate action?

a. Determine if the procedure had been fully explained by the physician.
b. Seek clarification of the grown daughter's concern.
c. Contact the physician to tell him of the grown daughter's concern.
d. Contact the on-duty chaplain for an ethical consult.

11. The physician performs the peritoneal tap but immediately following the procedure, the patient's blood pressure decreases significantly to 88/64 and breathing becomes more labored with a respiratory rate of 32 and a SpO_2 of 84 percent. Which of the following interventions would be most appropriate?

a. Deliver a 500 mL bolus of normal saline IV and assist breathing with a bag-valve-mask (BVM) at 100 percent oxygen.
b. Deliver 250 mL of albumin IV and assist breathing with a bag-valve-mask (BVM) at 100 percent oxygen.
c. Deliver a 500 mL bolus of normal saline IV and apply noninvasive positive pressure ventilation.
d. Deliver 250 mL of albumin IV and apply noninvasive positive pressure ventilation.

12. The patient is transferred to the intensive care unit where he is intubated and placed on mechanical ventilation. The daughter, in consultation with the tribal elders, elects to withdraw support. The daughter requests that a tribal drummer be allowed to drum and sing as her parent dies. A nurse coworker expresses concern regarding the perceived noise and disruption caused by the singing and drumming. Which of the following would be the most appropriate response to the coworker?

a. "We will have the ceremony outside in the garden."
b. "Don't you understand what the ceremony means to them?"
c. "What concerns do you have about the ceremony?"
d. "The physician has approved the ceremony in the room."

SCENARIO 4

A patient is admitted to the ICU with a diagnosis of meningococcemia. The patient arrives in the ICU intubated, ventilated, and requiring vasoactive drips to maintain blood pressure. Both parents are waiting in the adjacent waiting room. The following three questions relate to this scenario.

13. The nurse's initial assessment indicates that the patient has moderate levels of stability. The nurse goes to the waiting room and initially speaks with the parents regarding their child's condition. The parents' initial questions center on their child's survival over the next couple of hours. Which of the following statements would be most appropriate for the nurse to make?

a. "I hear your concerns, but I need more information before I can address them."
b. "The physician will be talking with you shortly and will tell you all that you need to know."
c. "I can arrange for a chaplain or your personal spiritual guide to meet with you."
d. "The patient is stabilizing, but we don't really know what will happen over the next couple of days."

14. The patient's condition improves with antibiotic therapy, but the patient remains sedated and on the ventilator. The vasoconstriction and purpura common with meningococcemia are resolving. The nurse elects to bathe the patient and asks the parents if they wish to assist. They refuse and suddenly say that they must leave the room while the bath is being completed. Which of the following is the most appropriate response by the nurse?
a. Discuss the rationale for providing the bath.
b. Insist that they provide help with the bath.
c. Provide the parents with an excuse to leave.
d. Ask about care they would like to provide.

15. The patient recovers quickly and the physician makes the decision to extubate and asks that it be done immediately. The patient is awake, responsive, and cooperative. Which of the following is the most appropriate action?
a. Describe the extubation process to the patient.
b. Immediately extubate the patient.
c. Administer a sedative/hypnotic to calm the patient.
d. Contact the parents to obtain consent.

SCENARIO 5

A flight nurse arrives at a referring hospital to accept a patient with burns for air medical transport to a burn center 100 miles away. The patient was caught on the second story of a house fire and has been burned over anterior portions of the lower extremities and up to the anterior mid-chest. Blood pressure has remained stable. The following four questions relate to this scenario.

16. On initial assessment, the nurse notes that the patient had just been intubated and moved from the ambulance stretcher to the ED stretcher. While assessing the airway, the nurse notes that there are no breath sounds over the chest and there is gurgling in the left upper abdomen with each compression of the bag-valve-mask (BVM) device. Which of the following actions would be the most appropriate?
a. Call for a STAT chest X-ray and check tube placement.
b. Extubate and reventilate with a bag-valve-mask (BVM) device.
c. Attach a capnography device and assess for color change.
d. Extubate and immediately reintubate the patient.

17. The nurse estimates that the patient's total body surface area (TBSA) with partial and full thickness burns equals approximately 25 percent. The nurse uses the Parkland formula to estimate the amount of IV fluid the patient will need during the first 24 hours of resuscitation. Which of the following is the correct formula that is multiplied by the TBSA with partial and full thickness burns to estimate the amount of IV fluid needed?
    a. 4 ml × kilograms of body weight
    b. 2 ml × kilograms of body weight
    c. 4 ml × pounds of body weight
    d. 2 ml × pounds of body weight

18. While completing a secondary assessment of the patient, the nurse notes that the right thigh is swollen and tight to touch. Upon closer examination, the nurse notes a small angulation of the thigh. Which of the following actions is the most appropriate?
    a. Splint the leg in the position found.
    b. Obtain an X-ray of the leg.
    c. Apply a Hare traction splint.
    d. Ask for physician confirmation.

19. As the nurse prepares to load the patient into the aircraft, the patient's parent asks about a burn center that is 150 miles in the other direction, but within easy driving distance of their home. The nurse knows that both burn centers are essentially equivalent in services. Which of the following is the nurse's most appropriate response?
    a. "Would it be better for you to transfer to the second hospital?"
    b. "We are already expected to arrive at the first hospital."
    c. "Are you concerned about the care at the first hospital?"
    d. "I will call to change the transfer to the second hospital."

SCENARIO 6

A patient is admitted to the ED with substantial chest pain that radiates to the left arm and neck, difficulty breathing, nausea, and vomiting. The symptoms have been present for 2 hours. In answers to questions, the patient states that there is no history of cardiac disease in the patient or immediate family. The following three questions relate to this scenario.

20. As part of the initial assessment, which of the following initial nursing actions would be most appropriate?
    a. Ask the patient's spouse about symptom onset.
    b. Attach a cardiac monitor and pulse oximetry to the patient.
    c. Assess airway, breathing, and circulation.
    d. Provide supplemental oxygen via a nonrebreather mask.

21. Ten minutes later, the patient's cardiac monitor alarms, displaying wide complex tachycardia. Finding no signs of spontaneous breathing or circulation, the nurse begins cardiopulmonary resuscitation and activates the

ED code team. The physician's first order is to administer amiodarone, 300 mg IV. Which of the following actions is most appropriate for the recorder nurse?

a. Repeat the order out loud.
b. Suggest epinephrine, 1 mg IV.
c. Suggest immediate defibrillation.
d. Ask for dose clarification.

22. The patient's spouse insists on remaining in the room while the code proceeds. Which of the following interventions is most appropriate?

a. Ask another nurse to stay with the spouse.
b. Stay with the spouse and explain the code.
c. Escort the spouse to the unit quiet room.
d. Ask a family member to stay with the spouse.

SCENARIO 7

A patient is admitted to the post anesthesia care unit (PACU) following a femoral-popliteal bypass graft to the right leg. A heparin drip is currently running at 1,000 units per hour. The patient is awake and following commands and is scheduled to be moved to the surgical unit within the next 30 minutes. The following three questions relate to this scenario.

23. The PACU nurse receives a report from the laboratory that the patient's aPTT is 21 seconds. Which of the following interventions is most appropriate?

a. Contact the surgeon for heparin adjustment orders.
b. Assess the patient's extremity for signs of ischemia.
c. Adjust the heparin drip per standing orders.
d. Contact the laboratory for a STAT aPTT redraw.

24. Just prior to calling report and transferring the patient to the surgical unit, the nurse conducts a final assessment of the patient. The patient is awake, alert, and answering questions appropriately. When questioned, the patient reports a loss of sensation and increased pain in the operative leg. The nurse is unable to locate the distal pulses in the affected extremity and notes that it is "dusky" when compared to the opposite leg. Which of the following is the most appropriate initial intervention?

a. Call for a STAT aPTT.
b. Contact the house supervisor.
c. Call report to the surgical unit.
d. Contact the attending surgeon.

25. The surgeon has determined that the graft has occluded and orders a return to surgery, in an attempt to open the graft. Discussing the return to surgery, the nurse notes that the patient is concerned about surviving a second surgery but understands its necessity if the extremity is to remain viable. As the patient is being returned to surgery, the patient requests a brief oppor-

tunity to talk with spouse and children, who are in the waiting room. Which of the following would be the most appropriate intervention?

a. Allow the patient a couple of minutes of visitation.
b. Contact the surgeon to talk with the family.
c. Disregard the patient's request for the visitation.
d. Explain the need for urgency in getting to the operating room.

ANSWER KEY AND RATIONALES TO ACUTELY AND CRITICALLY ILL ADULT PATIENT SAMPLE QUESTIONS

1. Answer a

Because of the types of injury, the patient will initially be highly vulnerable and fragile. The nurse's most appropriate initial task is to use clinical judgment in monitoring the patient for changes that could threaten the patient's physiological stability, such as inadequate ventilation and hemodynamic instability. In choice b, locating the patient's family and contacting the physician are important; however, they do not address the patient's characteristics of high vulnerability and low stability. In choice c, given the respiratory injuries identified and the patient's characteristics of high vulnerability and low stability, ensuring adequate ventilation is important. Locating the patient's family does not address the patient's characteristics of high vulnerability and low stability. In choice d, given the potential for bleeding and hemodynamic instability associated with pelvic fractures and the patient's characteristics of high vulnerability and low stability, monitoring for hemodynamic instability is important. Contacting the physician does not address the patient's characteristics of high vulnerability and low stability.

REFERENCES

Curley, M. A. Q. (1998). Patient-Nurse Synergy: Optimizing Patients' Outcomes. *American Journal of Critical Care* 7(1): 64–72.
Markey, D. W. (2001). Applying the Synergy Model: Clinical Strategies. *Critical Care Nurse* 21(3): 72–76.

2. Answer d

Allowing the patient to determine who visits him incorporates the nurse characteristics of advocacy/moral agency, caring practice, and response to diversity. Advocacy/moral agency represents the willingness of the nurse to work on the patient's behalf and allow deviations from the rules. Caring practice is demonstrated by the nurse's understanding of the patient's needs and allowing the patient to determine what is best. Response to diversity is illustrated by the nurse's sensitivity to age and gender considerations when dealing with the patient and realizing why the requests are being made. The patient is also exhibiting a willingness and ability to participate in decision making. In choice a, simply citing the visiting "rules" does not take into account the patient's capacity and ability to make such decisions and ignores response to diversity and ability to participate in decision making. In choice b, ignoring the patient's capacity and ability to make decisions regarding who visits him and discussing the issue with a chaplain does not represent the concerns of the patient and ignores response to diversity. In choice c, ignoring the patient's capacity and ability to make decisions regarding who visits him and discussing the issue with the patient's parents may meet their needs, but does not represent the concerns of the patient and ignores response to diversity.

REFERENCES

Curley, M. A. Q. (1998). Patient-Nurse Synergy: Optimizing Patients' Outcomes. *American Journal of Critical Care* 7(1): 64–72.
Kaplow, R. (2003). AACN Synergy Model for Patient Care: A Framework to Optimize Outcomes. *Critical Care Nurse* 23(Suppl. 1): 27–30.

3. Answer b

In this situation, the patient is moderately vulnerable and moderately stable as indicated by his ability to breathe and cough. Applying a 100 percent nonrebreather oxygen mask will meet the patient's immediate needs and address both vulnerability and stability. Clinical judgment will then allow the nurse to determine which course of action is the most appropriate to follow. In choice a, although the patient may ultimately need intubation, further information will be needed before asking for an immediate intubation. The patient is moderately vulnerable and moderately stable as indicated by his ability to breathe and cough. The patient has become unpredictable with the onset of the new symptoms. The nurse characteristic of clinical judgment is required to make this decision. In choice c, a nebulizer treatment will not affect the patient's vulnerability and stability. Again, the nurse characteristic of clinical judgment is required to make this decision and is based on the patient's condition and how likely the treatment will improve the patient's condition. In choice d, administering an antibiotic dose early will not affect the patient's vulnerability and stability. Again, the nurse characteristic of clinical judgment is required to make this decision and is based on the patient's condition and how likely the treatment will improve the patient's condition.

REFERENCES

Curley, M. A. Q. (1998). Patient-Nurse Synergy: Optimizing Patients' Outcomes. *American Journal of Critical Care* 7(1): 64–72.
Markey, D. M. (2001). Applying the Synergy Model: Clinical Strategies. *Critical Care Nurse* 21(3): 72–76.

4. Answer b

The patient's resiliency and resource availability is moderate in that the history of bronchitis is affecting his ability to wean and has already failed several attempts. Alternating periods of rest and activity over several days will increase the patient's endurance and strength. The nurse uses clinical judgment in evaluating the patient's response to the rest and activity and can modify the plan in accordance. In addition, the nurse will also assess the patient's readiness and ability to wean before the next attempt is made. In choice a, the patient's resiliency and resource availability are moderate in that the history of bronchitis is affecting his ability to wean. While stimulating a patient to assist with weaning is important during the actual weaning, adequate patient rest is required prior to the successful weaning. The nurse uses clinical judgment in evaluating both the patient's readiness and ability to wean. In choice c, although mental attitude is an important component in any physical accomplishment, encouragement is not the most helpful at this time. The patient's resiliency and resource availability is moderate in that the history of bronchitis is affecting his ability to wean. The patient will need both rest and activity, in addition to encouragement, to develop the strength to wean. The nurse uses clinical judgment evaluating both the patient's readiness and ability to wean. In choice d, as with mental attitude, rest is an important component in any physical accomplishment. However, sedatives tend to accumulate and may prevent the patient from participating in the activity needed to develop the strength to wean. The patient's resiliency and resource availability are moderate in that the history of bronchitis is affecting his ability to wean. The patient will need both rest and activity, in addition to encouragement, to develop the strength to wean. The nurse uses clinical judgment evaluating both the patient's readiness and ability to wean.

REFERENCES

Curley, M. A. Q. (1998). Patient-Nurse Synergy: Optimizing Patients' Outcomes. *American Journal of Critical Care* 7(1): 64–72.

Markey, D. M. (2001). Applying the Synergy Model: Clinical Strategies. *Critical Care Nurse* 21(3): 72–76.

5. Answer b

The patient has not had nutrition in several days and therefore is vulnerable with few inherent nutritional resources. Enteral nutrition is the correct answer because the nurse knows, using clinical inquiry, that if the gut works, it should be used. The naso-duodenal tube is easily placed and can provide the nutrients the patient will need. In choice a, although parental nutrition is effective in delivering nutrition, the most effective means is via the GI tract, if it is functional. In addition, the PICC line would require the insertion of a device that could provide a locus of infection. In choice c, although parental nutrition is effective in delivering nutrition, the most effective means is via the GI tract, if it is functional. In addition, the CVC would require the insertion of a device that could provide a locus of infection and place the risk of perforating the lung. In choice d, enteral nutrition is appropriate because if the gut works, it should be used. However, a PEG tube would require a surgical incision and is usually reserved for long-term support and not the correct answer, in this context.

REFERENCES

Markey, D. M. (2001). Applying the Synergy Model: Clinical Strategies. *Critical Care Nurse* 21(3): 72–76.
Trujillo, E. B., M. K. Robinson, and D. O. Jacobs. (2001). Feeding Critically Ill Patients: Current Concepts. *American Journal of Critical Care* 21(4): 60–69.

6. Answer c

The patient is highly vulnerable and has low resiliency immediately after being extubated. Using clinical inquiry, the nurse knows that patients who are intubated for as short as 24 hours exhibit difficulty in swallowing and may aspirate when resuming oral feeding. As this aspiration may be a significant cause of iatrogenic pneumonia, the nurse realizes that collaboration with speech therapy to evaluate the patient for swallowing difficulties may prevent an aspiration pneumonia that could extend the patient's hospitalization. In choice a, while possibly needing strengthening exercise to increase endurance, the patient's respiratory status is highly vulnerable, with low resiliency immediately after being extubated. Although collaboration is important, physical therapy would be delayed until the patient has a stable respiratory status.

In choice b, while probably needing assistance in coping with activities of daily living, the patient's respiratory status is highly vulnerable, with low resiliency immediately after being extubated. Although collaboration is important, occupational therapy would be delayed until the patient has a stable respiratory status. In choice d, while needing ongoing assessment and support for nutritional issues, the patient's respiratory status is highly vulnerable, with low resiliency immediately after being extubated. Although collaboration is important, nutritional assessment would be delayed until the patient has a stable respiratory status.

REFERENCE

Annis, T. D. (2002). The Interdisciplinary Team Across the Continuum of Care. *Critical Care Nurse* 22(5): 76–79.

7. Answer d

The patient's condition, coupled with the spouse's lack of understanding, makes the patient highly complex with impaired resource availability and ability to participate in care. The nurse uses systems thinking and collaboration to meet the spouse's stated concerns by contacting case management or social work for an evaluation of the couple's situation. Based on that evaluation, options can be developed that may meet both the patient's and the spouse's needs. In choice a, the patient's condition, coupled with the spouse's lack of understanding, makes the patient highly complex with impaired resource availability and ability to participate in care. Grown children may be able to assist with care, but given the complexity of the situation and lack of knowledge regarding the feasibility of this, home nursing consult would be a more appropriate answer. In choice b, although providing reassurance and information regarding wound care are helpful, they do not meet the stated needs of the spouse. The patient is highly complex and requires active intervention with additional resources if the patient and spouse are to successfully manage his discharge to home. In choice c, consulting with the patient's insurance carrier assumes that there is no other alternative to the complexity of the situation. The nurse is not usually in a position to spend a significant amount of time identifying alternatives. Case management and social work are conversant with the various alternatives and can provide such service to the patient and the nurse.

REFERENCES

Annis, T. D. (2002). The Interdisciplinary Team Across the Continuum of Care. *Critical Care Nurse* 22(5): 76–79.

Kaplow, R. (2003). AACN Synergy Model for Patient Care: A Framework to Optimize Outcomes. *Critical Care Nurse* 23(Suppl. 1): 27–30.

8. Answer a

Assessing the patient for signs and symptoms of heart failure reflects the nurse's clinical judgment and caring practices. Given the situation, the nurse understands that due to the recent CABG, the patient has decreased resiliency and increased vulnerability. Stability is also questionable, given the symptoms that the patient reports. An assessment will help establish whether the patient's symptoms are related to heart failure or simply fatigue and deconditioning. In choice b, consulting an occupational therapist would certainly be appropriate if the patient was simply fatigued and deconditioned. However, the issue of patient stability must be addressed before the home health nurse contemplates a referral. This can only be accomplished by a patient assessment. In choice c, contacting the physician for readmit orders without performing an actual assessment is premature. The patient may, in fact, need to be readmitted but until the home health nurse completes an assessment, there are no data to support that assumption. In choice d, arranging for the patient's grown son to provide daily help may be appropriate if the patient was simply fatigued and deconditioned. However, the issue of patient stability must be addressed before the home health nurse contemplates such an arrangement. This can only be accomplished by a patient assessment.

REFERENCES

Curley, M. A. Q. (1998). Patient-Nurse Synergy: Optimizing Patients' Outcomes. *American Journal of Critical Care* 7(1): 64–72.

Markey, D. W. (2001). Applying the Synergy Model: Clinical Strategies. *Critical Care Nurse* 21(3): 72–76.

9. Answer c

The patient described is highly vulnerable, unstable, and complex. However, without an assessment of the patient, stability and predictability are unknown. These factors must be assessed to determine the most appropriate placement of the patient. The nurse will use clinical judgment and systems thinking to assess the patient and make a determination of patient stability, in conjunction with the appropriateness of the assigned unit. If stable, the patient may remain in the ACU. If unstable, the patient may require stabilization and immediate transfer to the ICU. In choice a, code status determination is important, especially with a patient as complex as this. However, the nurse will need to initially focus on the patient's stability. This focus must start with an assessment of the patient. In choice b, although the patient's history may indicate a potential for transfer to an ICU, an initial assessment must be completed to identify whether or not the patient is stable. If stable, the patient may remain in the ACU. If unstable, the patient may require stabilization and immediate transfer to the ICU. In choice d, contacting the physician for orders without performing an actual assessment and establishing the stability of the patient is premature. The patient will eventually need orders, but the initial priority is to determine stability.

REFERENCE

Markey, D. W. (2001). Applying the Synergy Model: Clinical Strategies. *Critical Care Nurse* 21(3): 72–76.

10. Answer b

Asking for clarification from the grown daughter addresses both her resource availability and her ability to participant in decision making as a surrogate for her parent. Information from this interaction will assist the nurse using advocacy, caring practices, and response to diversity to assess the grown daughter's level of comprehension and understanding. In choice a, although determining if the procedure has been fully explained to the grown daughter is helpful, it is more important to determine what the grown daughter understands about the explanation and the procedure. Simply explaining something doesn't mean it was necessarily understood. In choice c, contacting the physician would be most appropriate *after* a discussion with the grown daughter and an understanding of her concerns, level of comprehension, and understanding. In choice d, the duty chaplain may be able to provide support for the daughter, but may not be able to assess the daughter's level of comprehension and understanding related to the procedure, thus addressing her concerns.

REFERENCE

McGaffic, C. (2001). The Synergy Model as a Foundation for Ethical Practice. *AACN News* 9: 6.

11. Answer a

The patient has become unstable and vulnerable with little resiliency to compensate for the drop in blood pressure and increasing difficulty in ventilation and oxygenation. By using a normal saline bolus instead of the albumin, the nurse utilizes both clinical judgment and clinical inquiry. The nurse will also utilize collaboration with the respiratory care provider in assisting the patient with ventilation using a BVM rather than the more complicated noninvasive positive pressure ventilation. In choice b, although albumin may increase the blood pressure, initial resuscitation with crystalloid solution is always the initial therapy to treat low blood pressure. Using a BVM rather than the more complicated noninvasive positive pressure ventilation for the initial stabilization of ventilation is more appropriate. In choice c, initial resuscitation with crystalloid solution is always the initial therapy to treat low blood pressure. Using a BVM rather than the more complicated noninvasive positive pressure ventilation for the initial stabilization of ventilation is more appropriate. In choice d, although albumin may increase the blood pressure, initial resuscitation with crystalloid solution is always the initial therapy to treat low blood pressure. Using a BVM rather than the more complicated noninvasive positive pressure ventilation for the initial stabilization of ventilation is more appropriate.

REFERENCES

Curley, M. A. Q. (1998). Patient-Nurse Synergy: Optimizing Patients' Outcomes. *American Journal of Critical Care* 7(1): 64–72.

Marino, P. (1998). *The ICU Book* 2nd ed. (pp. 221–222). Baltimore, MD: Williams & Wilkins.

12. Answer c

The daughter has requested a ceremony that is unique to their culture and which she believes is necessary for her parent's passage into death. The daughter is using her available resources to meet a perceived need. She is also engaged in decision making regarding her parent's care. The nurse addresses the situation by recognizing that the coworker apparently does not understand the meaning of the request to the daughter and patient. Using both moral advocacy and caring practices, the nurse works on behalf of the daughter and patient's rights and stated needs. The nurse also utilizes response to diversity and clinical inquiry to acknowledge and try to understand the coworker's concerns. This also provides an opportunity for the nurse to act as a facilitator of learning by providing education to the coworker regarding the specific cultural issues. In choice a, accepting the coworker's concerns as a valid excuse to prevent the completion of the ceremony in the presence of the patient removes the reason to have the ceremony in the first place. There may be alternative methods of completing the ceremony, but away from the patient is not one of them. The nurse is not acting as an advocate and is exhibiting low levels of response to diversity. In choice b, the tone of the response does nothing to explore the coworker's concerns and may be construed as an "attack" by the coworker. In fact, such a response may alienate the coworker from both the nurse and other patients of the same culture as the daughter and her parent. Here, again, the nurse is exhibiting low levels of response to diversity. In choice d, using the physician's order to deflect the coworker's concern does nothing to explore the meaning behind the comment. Blindly following orders does not take into account the uniqueness of each person's experience and may prevent an exploration of the comments and further education of the coworker regarding specific cultural issues.

REFERENCES

Kaplow, R. (2003). AACN Synergy Model for Patient Care: A Framework to Optimize Outcomes. *Critical Care Nurse* 23(Suppl. 1): 27–30.
McGaffic, C. (2001). The Synergy Model as a Foundation for Ethical Practice. *AACN News* 9: 6.

13. Answer d

The patient's condition is extremely unpredictable, as is the situation in which the parents find themselves. Meningococcemia can, and frequently will, lead to death or permanent disability. With rapid treatment, recovery can be complete, without sequela. The nurse uses clinical judgment, based on experience, and clinical inquiry, based on knowledge of the disease, to help the parents understand the complexities of treatment. As a facilitator of learning, the nurse presents the information in short, succinct bits that are easily absorbed. The nurse also understands that the stress of the situation may require that the same information be repeated multiple times before the parents absorb and accept it. In choice a, given the seriousness of the situation, the nurse has heard all that needs to be heard regarding the parents' immediate concern. The parents want to know if their child will survive and they are looking to the nurse to answer this extremely basic question. In choice b, the nurse is in the closest contact with the patient and can provide an up-to-date assessment of the current condition. Although the physician may be able to provide information as to the long-term prognosis, the nurse should fulfill this function for the patient's immediate condition. In choice c, although collaboration with a chaplain or spiritual advisor may be beneficial, it will not meet the parent's stated questions regarding survival. This type of information may only be obtained from the nurse or physician.

REFERENCES

Barkin, R. M., and P. Rosen, eds. (1999). *Emergency Pediatrics: A Guide to Ambulatory Care*, 5th ed. (pp. 713–714). St. Louis, MO: Mosby, Inc.

Curley, M. A. Q. (1998). Patient-Nurse Synergy: Optimizing Patients' Outcomes. *American Journal of Critical Care* 7(1): 64–72.

Markey, D. M. (2001). Applying the Synergy Model: Clinical Strategies. *Critical Care Nurse* 21(3): 72–76.

14. Answer d

By refusing and suddenly leaving the room, the parents have implicitly stated that they are not willing to participate in care to the level of bathing the patient. Utilizing response to diversity, the nurse recognizes this fact. However, the nurse also demonstrates caring practices to determine if there is any activity that the parents would feel comfortable providing for their child. This action gives them an opportunity to determine for themselves how they would like to participate in the care of their child. In choice a, by refusing to participate and suddenly leaving the room, the parents have implicitly stated that they are not willing to assist in bathing the patient. Discussing the rationale for the bath does not acknowledge their discomfort or unwillingness to be involved in the patient's care. The family is demonstrating a lack of willingness to participate in care of the patient. In choice b, insisting that they assist with the bath ignores the parents' desires. Ignoring their wishes implies a lack of respect on the part of the nurse and may even cause them to become hostile toward the nurse. In choice c, providing an excuse for the parents to leave ("I'll bet you're hungry"), allows them to avoid assisting with the bath. However, the nurse also loses the opportunity to determine with what tasks they would like to assist. With this response, the nurse is not attempting to increase family participation in care.

REFERENCE

Kaplow, R. (2003). AACN Synergy Model for Patient Care: A Framework to Optimize Outcomes. *Critical Care Nurse* 23(Suppl. 1): 27–30.

15. Answer a

The patient is moderately resilient, is moderately stable, and can actively partic-ipate in care. The patient is cooperative and needs to understand what "extuba-tion" means. The nurse uses clinical judgment, caring practices, and facilitation of learning to provide the patient with information regarding the extubation ex-perience. The patient will need to know how extubation will affect breathing and what sensations may be experienced. Understanding what activities are required immediately after extubation (coughing, breathing deeply) and how they impact ventilation and oxygenation will have a significant impact on the patient's con-tinued cooperation. In choice b, extubation of the patient without any patient preparation ignores both the need and consequences of not discussing the proce-dure with the patient. The patient's assistance at both the actual extubation and subsequent pulmonary hygiene is highly desirable, particularly with a patient who is alert and cooperative. In choice c, although a sedative/hypnotic may be ap-propriate for an agitated patient, it is not appropriate for this scenario. Adminis-tering a sedative would demonstrate a low level of clinical judgment. If a patient is alert and cooperative, they should be given information regarding anticipated procedures. In addition, they must be educated as to how their assistance can im-prove the outcome. In choice d, extubation is a medical decision that the physi-cian will make, based on the patient's condition. Although notifying the patient's parents is important, their consent is not required for extubation.

REFERENCES

Kaplow, R. (2003). AACN Synergy Model for Patient Care: A Framework to Optimize Outcomes. *Critical Care Nurse* 23(Suppl. 1): 27–30.
McGaffic, C. (2001). The Synergy Model as a Foundation for Ethical Practice. *AACN News* 9: 6.

16. Answer b

The patient is highly vulnerable and minimally stable because of the compromised airway. The nurse uses clinical judgment and clinical inquiry in both assessing the patient and determining the appropriate interventions, by knowing and following current advanced cardiac life support (ACLS) guidelines. Following extubation, reventilation with a bag-valve-mask device is necessary to both ventilate and oxy-genate the patient, prior to another attempt at intubation. In choice a, a chest X-ray may help determine the placement of the tube, but the patient assessment has al-ready determined that the endotracheal tube is in the esophagus. Obtaining the chest X-ray will inappropriately delay the definitive treatment, which is extubation and reventilation with a bag-valve-mask device. By selecting this response, the nurse would be demonstrating low levels of clinical judgment. The patient is ex-hibiting high levels of vulnerability and is unstable. In choice c, a capnography de-vice may help confirm the initial assessment of endotracheal tube displacement, but it will also inappropriately delay the definitive treatment, which is extubation and reventilation with a bag-valve-mask device. In choice d, absence of breath sounds and gurgling in the left upper quadrant of the abdomen indicates placement of the endotracheal tube in the esophagus. Although extubation is appropriate, the patient must be reventilated for at least 30 seconds prior to reintubation. In addition, intubation is not likely to be within a nurse's scope of practice.

REFERENCES

Curley, M. A. Q. (1998). Patient-Nurse Synergy: Optimizing Patients' Outcomes. *American Journal of Critical Care* 7(1): 64–72.
Markey, D. W. (2001). Applying the Synergy Model: Clinical Strategies. *Critical Care Nurse* 21(3): 72–76.

17. Answer a

The Parkland formula calculates the amount of IV fluid a burn victim will require over the first 24 hours from the time of injury. The formula is 4 ml × kilograms of body weight × TBSA partial and full thickness burns. The patient is vulnerable to the complications related to the burns. Although initially stable, given the age and percent of partial and full thickness burns, the patient is also highly complex. The nurse uses both clinical judgment and systems thinking in calculating the IV fluid rate according to the Parkland formula. The nurse understands that inadequate volume resuscitation may lead to hypovolemia, shock, and, ultimately, renal failure and systemic inflammatory response syndrome (SIRS). In choice b, the Parkland formula utilizes 4 ml (rather than 2 ml) × kilograms of body weight × TBSA partial and full thickness burns, to determine the amount of IV fluid needed over the first 24 hours. In choice c, the Parkland formula is 4 ml × kilograms (rather than pounds) of body weight × TBSA partial and full thickness burns, to determine the amount of IV fluid needed over the first 24 hours. In choice d, the Parkland formula is 4 ml (rather than 2 ml) × kilograms (rather than pounds of body weight) × TBSA partial and full thickness burns, to determine the amount of IV fluid needed over the first 24 hours.

REFERENCES

Curley, M. A. Q. (1998). Patient-Nurse Synergy: Optimizing Patients' Outcomes. *American Journal of Critical Care* 7(1): 64–72.
Danks, R. R. (2003). Burn Management: A Comprehensive Review of Epidemiology and Treatment of Burn Victims. *Journal of Emergency Medical Services* 28: 118–141.

18. Answer c

Because of the additional trauma to the right leg, the patient has become more vulnerable and complex and less resilient. Burns complicated by trauma become much more difficult to manage. The nurse uses clinical judgment and clinical inquiry to both assess the nature of the additional injury and determine its appropriate treatment. The nurse understands that stabilizing a long bone fracture will help relieve the muscle spasms and pain caused by the fracture. In addition, stabilization may well prevent fat emboli from being released from the fracture site during transport. In choice a, splinting the leg in position will neither relieve the pain caused by the muscle spasm nor prevent the fractured bone ends from overriding each other. A fractured femur will need to have some type of traction splint applied to stretch the muscles and overcome the spasms. The traction splint will also realign the ends of the fracture and relieve pain. In addition, stabilization with a traction splint may well prevent fat emboli from being released from the fracture site during transport. In choice b, obtaining an X-ray may help define the type of fracture but it will also delay the transfer of the patient to the burn center. Additionally, knowing the type of fracture will not usually affect the type of stabilization needed for transport. In choice d, consulting with the physician for confirmation of the nurse's assessment may delay the transport to the burn center. In addition, the physician's confirmation will not change the treatment.

REFERENCES

Curley, M. A. Q. (1998). Patient-Nurse Synergy: Optimizing Patients' Outcomes. *American Journal of Critical Care* 7(1): 64–72.
Markey, D. W. (2001). Applying the Synergy Model: Clinical Strategies. *Critical Care Nurse* 21(3): 72–76.

19. Answer a

The parent is expressing their desire to participate in decisions regarding care. Simply being closer to home may not be a valid reason to change the transfer. However, the nurse would ask the question to determine why the proximity to the burn center is important to the parent. The nurse would also use the question to explore the resource availability for the patient and family at the second hospital. In light of the patient's condition, the nurse would then evaluate the parent's stated needs utilizing clinical judgment, caring practices, and systems thinking to determine the appropriateness of the request. In choice b, the nurse's answer ignores the parent's request and the implied concerns and is therefore inappropriate. In choice c, although this answer may eventually get to the reason for the request, it does so in somewhat of a roundabout way. The nurse's question should address the stated concerns rather than making inferences as to the content of the concern. In choice d, the nurse's answer assumes that the single fact of the second burn center being closer to the patient's home overrides all other considerations, such as distance of transport and established relationship with the receiving physician. Further information needs to be gathered before making such a decision.

REFERENCES

Kaplow, R. (2003). AACN Synergy Model for Patient Care: A Framework to Optimize Outcomes. *Critical Care Nurse* 23(Suppl. 1): 27–30.

Markey, D. W. (2001). Applying the Synergy Model: Clinical Strategies. *Critical Care Nurse* 21(3): 72–76.

20. Answer d

Providing supplemental oxygen meets the patient's stated needs regarding difficulty in breathing. The patient is potentially highly vulnerable and minimally stable. The patient is also moderately predictable in that if the oxygen is not applied the difficulty in breathing will likely worsen. The nurse uses clinical judgment and advocacy in meeting the patient's stated need of difficulty in breathing by providing oxygen. Once breathing issues have been addressed, the assessment may proceed to addressing circulation. In addition, oxygen will help with the management of the chest pain. In choice a, the patient's spouse may provide additional information regarding the onset of symptoms, such as precipitating factors and the patient's reaction to the symptoms. However, this line of questioning does not address the patient's immediate stated need of difficulty in breathing. In choice b, one of the patient's immediate stated needs is difficulty in breathing. A cardiac monitor may provide information regarding the status of the patient's heart. The pulse oximetry may assist in assessing oxygenation status. However, neither action will intervene in the patient's most immediate need, shortness of breath. In choice c, assessment and intervention of any acutely ill patient should follow the "ABC" algorithm of airway, breathing, and circulation. Each is assessed sequentially and, if an abnormality is noted, interventions applied. The patient is speaking to the nurse so that the airway is known to be established and open. The patient reports difficulty in breathing. At this point, the nurse would stop the assessment and intervene. The initial intervention would be to provide supplemental oxygen and then reassess after a minute or so. Assessment of circulation could occur after the supplemental oxygen is applied.

REFERENCES

Curley, M. A. Q. (1998). Patient-Nurse Synergy: Optimizing Patients' Outcomes. *American Journal of Critical Care* 7(1): 64–72.

Markey, D. W. (2001). Applying the Synergy Model: Clinical Strategies. *Critical Care Nurse* 21(3): 72–76.

21. Answer c

The patient has minimal resiliency, is highly vulnerable, and has low levels of stability. Given the history and presentation of the patient, the cardiac rhythm is more likely ventricular tachycardia. Utilizing both clinical judgment and clinical inquiry, the nurse realizes that the most appropriate treatment would be immediate defibrillation. The nurse would make the suggestion using both collaboration and advocacy to optimize the patient outcome. In choice a, repeating an order out loud is an effective way to communicate understanding of the order and ensures that the understanding reflects the intent of the order. Unfortunately, the initial order is incorrect, both in context and dose. When faced with an order that is at odds with established care guidelines, the nurse must do more than simply repeat the order. This intervention is demonstrating low levels of clinical judgment and clinical inquiry as nationally established research-based guidelines are not being implemented. In choice b, using the ACLS guidelines, the nurse knows that epinephrine is more appropriate as the initial medication to be utilized in ventricular tachycardia. However, the most appropriate treatment would be immediate defibrillation. Epinephrine may increase the success of subsequent defibrillations, but the initial treatment should be immediate defibrillation. In choice d, utilizing the ACLS guidelines, the ordered dose of amiodarone (Cordarone®) is correct, but would be delivered only *after* the initial defibrillations and an initial dose of epinephrine. In this situation, the most appropriate treatment would be immediate defibrillation.

REFERENCES

American Heart Association. (2000). Guidelines 2000 for Cardiopulmonary Resuscitation and Emergency Cardiovascular Care. International Consensus on Science. *Circulation* 102(Suppl. 8).

Curley, M. A. Q. (1998). Patient-Nurse Synergy: Optimizing Patients' Outcomes. *American Journal of Critical Care* 7(1): 64–72.

Kaplow, R. (2003). AACN Synergy Model for Patient Care: A Framework to Optimize Outcomes. *Critical Care Nurse* 23(Suppl. 1): 27–30.

22. Answer b

Staying with the spouse and explaining the code addresses the spouse's need to participate in care, even if it is just by watching what is happening. The spouse's needs are highly complex at this time. In this example, the patient's care is relatively straightforward: airway, breathing, and circulation. The spouse's needs are primarily emotional and psychological, dealing with the potential death of a loved one. In addition, the spouse has few resources available to interpret what is occurring during the code and needs the nurse's knowledge and perspective. The nurse utilizes advocacy, caring practice, clinical inquiry, and facilitation of learning to meet the spouse's needs. In addition, the nurse utilizes clinical inquiry by knowing the current literature that addresses the issue of family presence during a code. In choice a, the initial nurse will have the most effective communication with the spouse because they have established a relationship, albeit a short one. The initial nurse will be the spouse's most effective guide to understanding what is happening during the code. Asking another nurse to stay with the spouse takes the initial nurse away from the spouse, forcing the spouse to establish a relation-ship with another nurse, this time in an even more stressful environment. In choice c, removing the spouse from the room ignores the spouse's stated request and need. Although some medical personnel may be uncomfortable with family members' presence during a code, nursing research supports their presence at the code as beneficial to the spouse, the patient, and the care providers. In choice d, asking family members to stay with the spouse may provide support for the spouse but does not address the process of what is happening with the code. The nurse loses a valuable opportunity to assist the spouse in understanding what is happening to the patient and provide emotional and psychological support.

REFERENCES

Kaplow, R. (2003). AACN Synergy Model for Patient Care: A Framework to Optimize Outcomes. *Critical Care Nurse* 23(Suppl. 1): 27–30.

MacLean, S. L., Guzzetta, C. E., White, C., Fontaine, D., Eichhorn, D. J., Meyers, T. A., and Désy, P. (2003). Family Presence During Cardiopulmonary Resuscitation and Invasive Procedures: Practices of Critical Care and Emergency Nurses. *American Journal of Critical Care* 12(3): 246–257.

McGaffic, C. (2001). The Synergy Model as a Foundation for Ethical Practice. *AACN News* 9: 6.

23. Answer c

The patient is highly vulnerable because of the recent surgery and, with regard to coagulation, has minimal resiliency. The patient's coagulation status is being con-trolled by the heparin drip. Using clinical judgment, the nurse understands that the aPTT is an index of coagulation and is tightly regulated after surgery to pre-vent the graft from clotting. An uncorrected aPTT may lead to clotting of the graft and ischemia of the entire limb. By implementing the standing orders, the nurse attempts to correct the aPTT in the most efficient manner possible. In choice a, contacting the surgeon for orders may take some time. The aPTT value indicates that the patient's coagulation status is unacceptable and any delay in addressing it could jeopardize the graft and cause ischemia. Standing orders are routine for surgeries such as described in this question and are utilized to allow the nurse to use clinical judgment in adjusting such drips. In choice b, the nurse has been pre-sented with an abnormal laboratory finding, which indicates that the patient's co-agulation status is unacceptable. Any delay in addressing it could jeopardize the graft and cause limb ischemia. Assessing the extremity may or may not yield ad-ditional information. The core issue of the question is that the aPTT needs to be corrected as soon as possible. Additional time taken to assess the extremity may delay such correction. In choice d, the initial aPTT indicates that the patient's co-agulation status is unacceptable. Requesting a "STAT redraw" would delay ad-justment of the heparin drip, which could jeopardize the graft and cause limb ischemia.

REFERENCE

Curley, M. A. Q. (1998). Patient-Nurse Synergy: Optimizing Patients' Outcomes. *American Journal of Critical Care* 7(1): 64–72.

24. Answer d

The patient has become minimally resilient, highly vulnerable, and minimally stable. Based on the patient's assessment, the nurse uses clinical judgment to determine that the graft has potentially clotted off. Without immediate intervention, the patient may lose the affected leg. The nurse utilizes collaboration in contacting the surgeon because the patient will likely require additional surgery. In choice a, based on the assessment the nurse realizes that the graft has potentially clotted off. Although a STAT aPTT may indeed be required, the surgeon should be notified first, so that a more detailed assessment of and intervention to preserve the extremity may be ordered. In choice b, the house supervisor will need to be made aware of the change in the patient's condition because it may affect the patient's placement after surgery. This intervention will be appropriate after the surgeon determines the treatment the patient requires. In choice c, the surgical unit will need to be notified of the change in the patient's condition because it may affect the patient's placement after surgery and may require the patient to be placed in another unit. This notification will assist the surgical unit in staffing and placement of other admissions on their unit. This intervention will be appropriate after the surgeon determines the treatment the patient requires.

REFERENCE

Kaplow, R. (2003). AACN Synergy Model for Patient Care: A Framework to Optimize Outcomes. *Critical Care Nurse* 23(Suppl. 1): 27–30.

25. Answer a

The patient and family are highly vulnerable because of the potentially life-altering emergency surgery that has to be undertaken. The emergent nature of the situation and decision to return to surgery make the patient and family minimally stable and highly complex. The patient has expressed full willingness to participate in care and decision making by verbalizing an understanding of the need for the surgery and making the decision to allow it to occur. The nurse uses both clinical judgment and advocacy in understanding the needs of the patient and family, in spite of the brief time delay that would ensure getting the patient to surgery. The nurse also uses caring practices to see that the patient's request is fulfilled. In choice b, the surgeon will need to talk with the family at some point to explain the surgery and its potential results. However, this intervention does not meet the patient's stated needs of talking with spouse and children. In choice c, the patient has made a specific request that needs to be addressed. The nurse may feel the need to disregard the request in the interest of getting the patient to the operating room as soon as possible. However, in doing so, the nurse ignores the established duty to be an advocate for both the patient and family and assist them in meeting their needs. In choice d, although there is certainly an "emergent" need to get to surgery as soon as possible, the patient has verbalized an understanding of the situation and made the decision that talking with the spouse and family is more important. The patient certainly has the right to make such a decision. The nurse should not attempt to advise against such a decision but should act as a facilitator so that the patient's (and family's) identified needs are met.

REFERENCE

McGaffic, C. (2001). The Synergy Model as a Foundation for Ethical Practice. *AACN News* 9: 6.

CHAPTER 19

THE ACUTELY AND CRITICALLY ILL PEDIATRIC PATIENT SAMPLE QUESTIONS

Deborah L. Bingaman, MS, RN, CPNP, CCNS
Roberta Kaplow, PhD, RN, CCNS, CCRN

INTRODUCTION

The following questions have been developed to provide examples of questions that integrate the pediatric patient and nurse characteristics of the AACN Synergy Model. The scenarios and questions in this chapter focus on acutely and critically ill pediatric patients in a variety of patient care settings. Each question is followed by four choices; one answer is best. An annotated key at the end of the questions provides the correct choice along with a rationale for why the other choices are not the best, based on the AACN Synergy Model.

1. A 3-year-old patient with epiglottitis is in the pediatric intensive care unit (PICU). Parents should be instructed to notify the health care professional if the child develops:
   a. Barking cough
   b. Hoarseness
   c. Bradycardia
   d. Muffled voice

2. You are caring for a patient in the PICU with severe acute exacerbation of asthma. Which of the following ABG results is consistent with this diagnosis?

	pH	pCO_2	pO_2	SaO_2	HCO_3
a.	7.50	30	78	96	19
b.	7.44	35	62	91	20
c.	7.38	38	58	88	21
d.	7.25	50	52	86	16

3. You are caring for a patient in the PICU on mechanical ventilation for pneumonia. The mother states, "The last time my son was on the breathing machine, the nurse caring for him came in and suctioned him every 2 hours." Which of the following is the best response?
   a. "Would you like me to suction your son?"
   b. "I will call the respiratory therapist to see if your son needs to be suctioned."
   c. "Routine suctioning is not recommended and can cause harm."
   d. "Do you feel I am not providing adequate care to your son?"

4. Which of the following diagnostic (ECG and chest X-ray, respectively) findings are consistent with a diagnosis of patent ductus arteriosus?
   a. Mild right ventricular hypertrophy; enlarged right ventricle
   b. Right atrial enlargement; pulmonary hypertension
   c. Left axis deviation; cardiomegaly
   d. Left ventricular hypertrophy; left atrial enlargement

5. A 3-year-old patient with a history of uncorrected tetralogy of Fallot is in the PICU with fever, headache, nausea, and vomiting. Which of the following diagnostic tests should the nurse prepare the patient for?
   a. Lumbar puncture
   b. Computed tomography
   c. CBC for white blood cell count
   d. Brain scan

SCENARIO 1

Questions 6 and 7 refer to the following scenario.

You are caring for a 3-month-old child in the PICU with congestive heart failure related to a large ventricular septal defect. The child developed tachypnea, increased work of breathing, nasal flaring, use of accessory muscles, and poor feeding at home. The child has been receiving digoxin at home to manage the congestive heart failure. Vital signs are within normal limits. Lab findings are as follows:

K   3.2
Mg 0.9
Ca 11.2

Digoxin level 1.5 (normal = < 2.2; toxic levels > 2–3.5)

6. The child develops bradycardia with rare new premature ventricular contractions, lethargy, vomiting, and diarrhea. Which of the following is indicated first?
   a. Collaborate with physician to administer digoxin-specific Fab antibody fragments.
   b. Notify the physician and withhold further digoxin administration.
   c. Provide bag-valve-mask ventilation and administer atropine 0.02 mg/kg.
   d. Administer a normal saline bolus of 20 ml/kg.

7. Two hours later, the child develops sustained ventricular tachycardia with a pulse. The patient is hypotensive and has signs of poor systemic perfusion. Which of the following is **NOT** indicated at this time?
   a. Synchronized cardioversion
   b. Digoxin-specific Fab antibody fragments (Digibind®)
   c. Propranolol (Inderal®) 0.01–0.15 mg/kg
   d. Procainamide (Pronestyl®) 10–15 mg/kg over 30 minutes

8. A 9-year-old with terminal cancer is admitted to the PICU with pneumonia. The parents seem to be denying the terminal nature of their child's condition. The child asks, "Am I dying?" The nurse's best response is:
   a. "Are you afraid of being separated from your parents?"
   b. "Would you like me to go get your parents?"
   c. "It is possible that you might die but we are doing everything we can to help you."
   d. "What is the worst thing about dying to you?"

9. A 2-year-old is admitted to the PICU from the emergency department status post motor vehicle crash with car seat failure; B/P = 90/50; HR = 150. Distal pulses are faint; capillary refill time = 4 seconds; skin is mottled and pale. Which of the following is indicated at this time?
   a. Transfusion of 2 units PRBCs
   b. Administration of 5% albumin, 20 ml/kg
   c. Administration of normal saline, 20 ml/kg
   d. Titration of dopamine from 5 mcg/kg/min

10. A 10-month-old child is admitted to the PICU with stridor, cough and hoarseness, mild fever, and two days of anorexia. This is suggestive of which of the following?
    a. Bronchiolitis
    b. Epiglottitis
    c. Bacterial pneumonia
    d. Laryngotracheobronchitis

11. A PICU nurse orientee is caring for an unconscious teenager with a head injury who is having frequent spikes in ICP. The preceptor observes the orientee neglecting to maintain a neutral, midline position of the patient's head. The preceptor should best correct the orientee by:
    a. Reassigning the orientee to a less unstable patient.
    b. Immediately repositioning the patient's head.
    c. Making a note in the nurse's orientation record.
    d. Directing the orientee to reposition the patient's head.

12. An 8-month-old former premature infant with chronic lung disease is trached and chronically vented. The infant has suffered a significant neurological insult after a severe episode of sepsis with meningitis. The PICU team has discussed withdrawing support. The cultural beliefs of the parents do not support this. The parents speak very little English. The nurse can best support the family by:

   a. Having a translator meet with the family to explain the infant's prognosis and obtain their input.

   b. Providing the family with literature in their language explaining the infant's current clinical situation.

   c. Working with a translator to evaluate the parents' understanding of the current clinical situation.

   d. Setting up a care conference with the PICU team and family and translator to discuss withdrawal of support.

13. A 3-week-old infant with Hypoplastic Left Heart Syndrome has undergone a heart transplant a week ago. The infant is stable and will be transferred to the step-down unit later today. In talking to the mother, the nurse discovers that she thinks the baby will only require immunosuppressive medications for a few months. The nurse should:

   a. Assess the mother's knowledge of the long-term care of her child after transplant.

   b. Report this information to the transplant social worker.

   c. Provide literature to the mother requiring the need for lifetime immunosuppression.

   d. Refer the mother back to the transplant team for clarification.

14. The PICU clinical practice committee has expressed an interest in participating in research and would like to replicate a skin care research protocol done in a smaller unit. The nursing staff has never done a research project before and is reluctant to participate. To facilitate this process, the committee nurses should:

   a. Initiate the process despite the staff concerns because they know that it is an easy protocol and the staff will pick it up easily.

   b. Introduce the steps of the research process through in-service meetings for all the staff members.

   c. Select a small group of staff nurses who want to participate and do not worry about the others.

   d. Limit participation in the research project to clinical practice committee members only.

15. A 3-year-old with a splenic injury status post MVA requires a blood transfusion for a decreasing hematocrit. The parents are Jehovah's Witnesses and refused to consent for the transfusion earlier in the day. They left the unit after being informed that a court order for the transfusion would be obtained. When they returned to the bedside later, they observe the blood infusing. They are angry and insist that the transfusion be stopped immediately. The nurse can best support the family by:

   a. Notifying hospital security to come and escort the family from the unit if necessary.

   b. Referring the family to the trauma social worker for counseling.

   c. Acknowledging the parents' religious beliefs while explaining the emergent need.

   d. Referring them to the ICU attending physician to discuss the problem.

16. A cardiologist has complained that most nurses in the ICU do not know how to care for a patient with a pacemaker after cardiac surgery and wants only certain nurses to care for these patients. Several nurses in the unit have formed a task force to evaluate the problem and develop a solution. Initially the nurses can best handle this problem by:
   a. Setting up mandatory pacemaker in-services for all unit nurses.
   b. Meeting with the cardiologist to discuss his specific concerns.
   c. Referring the cardiologist to the nurse manager to resolve this problem.
   d. Including pacemaker care as part of the annual competency review.

17. The ICU physicians have approached the PICU management regarding purchasing a new patient care monitoring system. The nursing manager has asked the clinical practice committee to spearhead this effort. The initial action by the clinical practice committee would be to:
   a. Contact sales representatives from various companies to send literature regarding their monitoring systems.
   b. Send questionnaires to other similar units to collect information regarding their current monitoring systems.
   c. Recommend developing a task force of physicians, nurses, the unit APN, the nurse manager, and other pertinent ancillary staff.
   d. Survey the unit staff regarding their likes and dislikes regarding the current monitoring system.

18. An 18-month-old status post near drowning is demonstrating decorticate posturing. The parents are excited to see their child moving his extremities. They insist that their child is trying to suck his thumb "like he used to." The nurse can best explain this type of neurological behavior from anoxic brain injury to the parents by:
   a. Providing the parents with written patient education materials.
   b. Having the PICU CNS meet with the parents.
   c. Setting up a patient care conference to discuss long-term prognosis.
   d. Taking the time to explain this behavior and evaluating their understanding.

SCENARIO 2

Questions 19–21 are based on the following information.
   A 12-year-old, 32 kg, is admitted to the ICU newly diagnosed diabetic with DKA.

Glucose	626	BP 88/50	U/O 50 ml/hour
Na	148	HR 128	
K	4.0	CRT >5 sec	

19. This patient is exhibiting what type of shock?
   a. Cardiogenic
   b. Septic
   c. Hypovolemic
   d. Anaphylactic

20. Initial fluid resuscitation for this patient should be as follows:
    a. 20 ml/kg NS over 1 hour, then replace remaining deficit over the next 24–48 hours.
    b. 20 ml/kg NS over 1 hour, then replace remaining deficit over the next 12–24 hours.
    c. 10 ml/kg LR over 1 hour, then replace remaining deficit over the next 24–48 hours.
    d. 10 ml/kg LR over 1 hour, then replace remaining deficit over the next 12–24 hours.

21. An insulin drip was started and 2 hours later the patient has the following labs and vital signs:

Glucose	246	BP 98/56	U/O 30 ml/hour
Na	132	HR 94	
K	3.4	CRT 3 sec	

Based on these findings, the IV fluids should change to:
    a. D5/ NS
    b. D10/.45 NS
    c. D5/.45 NS with KCL
    d. D10/.2 NS with KCL

22. An 8-month-old former premature infant who has been chronically ventilated since birth had a tracheostomy done 2 days ago. The parents have confided to the nurse that they will never be able to learn what they need to know to care for their child at home. They fear that their baby will never leave the hospital. Initially, the nurse can best approach helping this family overcome their fears by:
    a. Having the parents observe each step of care and gradually take over.
    b. Talking the family through site care as they do it the first time.
    c. Showing the family a video and then having them do the site care on their own.
    d. Giving the family written materials and then having them do the care on their own.

SCENARIO 3

Questions 23 and 24 are based on the following information.

A 2-year-old has been admitted to the ICU with a history of flu-like symptoms that initially improved. On the day of admission, the child became increasingly lethargic with recurrent fever and was very pale. In the ED, the following exam showed:

BP	74/46	O_2 sat 88% (room air)
HR	178	CRT >5 second
RR	48	

Cardiac auscultation reveals a gallop with a Grade III/VI murmur. Auscultation of the lungs reveals crackles.

23. This patient is exhibiting what kind of shock:
    a. Anaphylactic
    b. Hypovolemic
    c. Cardiogenic
    d. Septic

24. Initial management for this patient would include:
    a. Fluid resuscitation and corticosteroids
    b. Anticoagulation therapy and afterload reduction
    c. Inotropic support and afterload reduction
    d. Inotropic support and corticosteroids

25. A 3-year-old status post VSD closure with known elevated pulmonary artery pressures preoperatively returns to the ICU on the ventilator. Preoperative pulmonary pressures were near systemic. Vital signs are:

    PAP   48/18 mean 32   HR   110   BP   100/52

Two hours later, the patient is beginning to move around and cough. Vital signs are:

    PAP   58/22 mean 40   HR 168   BP   92/44

What ongoing precautions should the nurse take to prevent a pulmonary hypertensive crisis:
    a. Use lidocaine down the endotracheal tube before suctioning.
    b. Maintain adequate IV sedation before suctioning.
    c. Preoxygenate with 100 percent O_2 before suctioning.
    d. Hyperventilate the patient before suctioning.

ANSWER KEY AND RATIONALES TO ACUTELY AND CRITICALLY ILL PEDIATRIC PATIENT SAMPLE QUESTIONS

1. Answer d

Epiglottitis is a medical emergency characterized by severe airway obstruction caused by inflammation and swelling of the epiglottis, false cords, and aryepiglottic folds. The child often demonstrates a muffled voice and weak cough, in contrast to the barking cough and hoarseness seen in laryngotracheobronchitis. Other signs and symptoms include high fever, sore throat, drooling, and dysphagia. Swelling of the epiglottis produces signs of progressive airway obstruction including sternal retractions, tachycardia, and decreased breath sounds.

In this situation, the child is exhibiting high levels of vulnerability by being at high risk for a medical emergency. The child is vulnerable and unprotected. The parents are exhibiting moderate levels to participate in care, as they will be receiving information to assist in the care of their child. The nurse is exhibiting moderate levels as a facilitator of learning by incorporating the family's understanding into practice. The nurse is also exhibiting moderate levels of clinical judgment by demonstrating knowledge of clinically significant symptoms to be monitored.

REFERENCES

Curley, M. A. Q. (1998). Patient-Nurse Synergy: Optimizing Patients' Outcomes. *American Journal of Critical Care* 7(1): 64–72.

Hazinski, M. F. (1999). *Manual of Pediatric Critical Care.* St. Louis, MO: Mosby, Inc.

Kaplow, R. (2003). AACN Synergy Model for Patient Care: A Framework to Optimize Outcomes. *Critical Care Nurse* 23(Suppl. 1): 27–30.

2. Answer d

Severe acute exacerbation of asthma is characterized by a metabolic and respiratory acidosis. PH is below normal, pCO_2 will be elevated, SaO_2 is below normal, and pO_2 is below normal limits.

In this situation, the child is exhibiting high levels of vulnerability and is susceptible and fragile in the clinical state presented. The nurse is exhibiting moderate levels of clinical judgment by collecting and interpreting complex patient data and making clinical judgments based on a grasp of the big picture of the patient with a severe acute exacerbation of asthma.

REFERENCES

Curley, M. A. Q. (1998). Patient-Nurse Synergy: Optimizing Patients' Outcomes. *American Journal of Critical Care* 7(1): 64–72.

Hazinski, M. F. (1999). *Manual of Pediatric Critical Care* (p. 331). St. Louis, MO: Mosby, Inc.

Kaplow, R. (2003). AACN Synergy Model for Patient Care: A Framework to Optimize Outcomes. *Critical Care Nurse* 23(Suppl. 1): 27–30.

3. Answer c

Suctioning should be performed whenever there is evidence of accumulation of secretions or whenever there is a question of tube obstruction. This means that the need for suctioning must be determined individually; "routine" suctioning should not be performed. Unnecessary suctioning should not be performed and may cause mucosal damage and stimulate additional mucus production.

In this situation, the patient has a moderate level of vulnerability, being somewhat susceptible. The child has overcome pneumonia in the past but requires mechanical ventilation for another bout of pneumonia. The child also seems to be moderately stable, able to maintain a steady state for a period of time. The nurse in this situation, by selecting the best response, is demonstrating a Level 3 for clinical judgment. The nurse is making judgments based on an immediate grasp of the whole picture of the patient. The nurse demonstrated a Level 3 for caring practices by tailoring care based on individual patient needs. By choosing choice a, the nurse would not be individualizing care based on patient need nor basing care on the most recent evidence regarding suctioning. In choice b, the nurse is showing the ability to collaborate with one of the members of the multidisciplinary team. However, this response is not appropriate in this situation for two reasons. First, suctioning is a procedure that can be performed by the nurse. Second, there does not seem to be an indication for suctioning at the present time.

REFERENCES

Curley, M. A. Q. (1998). Patient-Nurse Synergy: Optimizing Patients' Outcomes. *American Journal of Critical Care* 7(1): 64–72.

Hazinski, M. F. (1999). *Manual of Pediatric Critical Care* (p. 324). St. Louis, MO: Mosby, Inc.

Kaplow, R. (2003). AACN Synergy Model for Patient Care: A Framework to Optimize Outcomes. *Critical Care Nurse* 23(Suppl. 1): 27–30.

4. Answer d

The findings in choice a are consistent with an atrial septal defect. Choice b is consistent with a ventricular septal defect. The findings in choice c are consistent with endocardial cushion defect.

In this situation, the patient is exhibiting moderate levels of vulnerability, being somewhat susceptible to problems given the cardiac condition described. The nurse demonstrated Level 3 clinical judgment by making decisions based on the immediate grasp of the whole picture for a common patient population. By understanding the pathophysiology of patent ductus arteriosus, the nurse can determine the correct ECG and radiologic findings associated with this disorder.

REFERENCES

Curley, M. A. Q. (1998). Patient-Nurse Synergy: Optimizing Patients' Outcomes. *American Journal of Critical Care* 7(1): 64–72.

Hazinski, M. F. (1999). *Manual of Pediatric Critical Care* (p. 221). St. Louis, MO: Mosby, Inc.

Kaplow, R. (2003). AACN Synergy Model for Patient Care: A Framework to Optimize Outcomes. *Critical Care Nurse* 23(Suppl. 1): 27–30.

5. Answer b

Children with uncorrected cyanotic cardiac disease can develop brain abscesses. Signs and symptoms of brain abscess formation can be extremely nonspecific.

The most common trio of symptoms include fever, headache, and focal neurologic abnormalities. Other signs and symptoms include nausea and vomiting or other signs of increased intracranial pressure. Health care team members must have a high index of suspicion when patients are at risk for the development of a brain abscess because these signs can be missed. A normal WBC is observed in many children with brain abscesses. The computed tomography is diagnostic for brain abscess and should be performed before lumbar puncture in any child with cyanotic heart disease presenting with fever, headache, and focal neurologic findings. Lumbar puncture is only performed if the CT scan is negative.

In this situation, the patient is highly vulnerable (Level 1), being susceptible and fragile with uncorrected cyanotic cardiac disease, a complication associated with the condition. The patient is manifesting clinically significant symptoms that require intervention. By selecting the correct response, the nurse is demonstrating Level 3 clinical judgment by making judgments regarding complications of a condition and knowledge of the diagnostic tests that are indicated. Further, moderate levels of clinical judgment are apparent from the nurse's collecting and interpreting complex patient data regarding the symptoms of brain abscesses. The nurse is demonstrating Level 3 as a facilitator of learning by developing an educational plan based on the data collected.

REFERENCES

Curley, M. A. Q. (1998). Patient-Nurse Synergy: Optimizing Patients' Outcomes. *American Journal of Critical Care* 7(1): 64–72.

Hazinski, M. F. (1999). *Manual of Pediatric Critical Care* (pp. 198–199, 201). St. Louis, MO: Mosby, Inc.

Kaplow, R. (2003). AACN Synergy Model for Patient Care: A Framework to Optimize Outcomes. *Critical Care Nurse* 23(Suppl. 1): 27–30.

6. Answer b

Serum digoxin levels should be interpreted with caution. Hypokalemia, hypomagnesemia, and hypercalcemia can aggravate digoxin cardiotoxicity even in the presence of "normal" serum digoxin levels. Presence of clinical symptoms should be interpreted more strongly than serum digoxin level alone. Digoxin-specific Fab antibody fragments should be administered to patients with malignant arrhythmias, hypotension, and poor systemic perfusion. Interventions c and d are not indicated at this time given the presented information.

In this situation, the child is demonstrating high levels of vulnerability and low levels of stability and resiliency. The child is highly susceptible and fragile, is labile, is having complications of therapy and the underlying cardiac condition, and is not demonstrating an ability to compensate for the heart failure. The nurse, by selecting the appropriate response, is demonstrating Level 3 clinical judgment. The nurse demonstrated an ability to get an immediate grasp on the whole picture for the patient and collect and interpret complex patient data.

REFERENCES

Curley, M. A. Q. (1998). Patient-Nurse Synergy: Optimizing Patients' Outcomes. *American Journal of Critical Care* 7(1): 64–72.

Hazinski, M. F. (1999). *Manual of Pediatric Critical Care* (pp. 121, 124). St. Louis, MO: Mosby, Inc.

Kaplow, R. (2003). AACN Synergy Model for Patient Care: A Framework to Optimize Outcomes. *Critical Care Nurse* 23(Suppl. 1): 27–30.

7. Answer a

Synchronized cardioversion should not be performed for ventricular tachycardia secondary to digoxin toxicity, because it may convert ventricular tachycardia into ventricular fibrillation or asystole. Propranolol or procainamide may be used to treat ventricular arrhythmias. Digoxin-specific Fab antibody fragments is now indicated because the child has a malignant arrhythmia secondary to digoxin toxicity.

In this situation, the child is demonstrating high levels of vulnerability and low levels of stability and resiliency. The child is highly susceptible, fragile, and labile as evidenced by the presence of a life-threatening arrhythmia. An incorrect intervention, in this case synchronized cardioversion, could have lethal consequences.

REFERENCES

Curley, M. A. Q. (1998). Patient-Nurse Synergy: Optimizing Patients' Outcomes. *American Journal of Critical Care* 7(1): 64–72.

Hazinski, M. F. (1999). *Manual of Pediatric Critical Care* (p. 125). St. Louis, MO: Mosby, Inc.

Kaplow, R. (2003). AACN Synergy Model for Patient Care: A Framework to Optimize Outcomes. *Critical Care Nurse* 23(Suppl. 1): 27–30.

8. Answer c

The child's parents are often the best people to talk to the child about death, but they will require assistance from the health care professional. A child's questions must be answer honestly while maintaining an element of hope. It is extremely important to clarify and then answer the child's question rather than the questions anticipated by the nurse or parent. The child may become angry if the perception is that the questions and concerns are being ignored or avoided. Parental separation is a fear associated with infancy. Choice d would be an appropriate response if the child stated "I don't want to die."

In this situation, the child is exhibiting high levels of vulnerability as evidenced by the presence of terminal cancer. The child is also demonstrating high levels of complexity due to the parents' inability to accept the terminal nature of their child's illness compounded with the physiologic condition of the child. The nurse is exhibiting Level 3 for caring practices by engaging with the patient as a unique individual in a compassionate manner. The nurse is also exhibiting Level 3 as a facilitator of learning by providing age-appropriate information to the child based on the question posed.

REFERENCES

Curley, M. A. Q. (1998). Patient-Nurse Synergy: Optimizing Patients' Outcomes. *American Journal of Critical Care* 7(1): 64–72.
Hazinski, M. F. (1999). *Manual of Pediatric Critical Care* (pp. 74–75). St. Louis, MO: Mosby, Inc.
Kaplow, R. (2003). AACN Synergy Model for Patient Care: A Framework to Optimize Outcomes. *Critical Care Nurse* 23(Suppl. 1): 27–30.

9. Answer c

The child is showing signs of late shock. Tachycardia is a nonspecific sign of distress and hypotension is a late sign of shock. Volume replacement is indicated. Colloids may cause sensitivity reactions and other complications. PRBCs and other blood products for replacement of blood loss or correction of coagulopathies may be required. Blood is ideal fluid replacement for fluid losses sustained by pediatric trauma victims who demonstrate evidence of hypovolemic shock despite two fluid boluses of crystalloid.

In this situation, the child is demonstrating high levels of vulnerability and low levels of stability and resiliency. The child is highly susceptible, fragile, and labile due to having signs of late shock. The nurse is demonstrating Level 3 clinical judgment by making clinical judgments based on the immediate grasp of the whole patient picture and by collecting and interpreting complex data.

REFERENCES

Chameides, L., Hazinski, M. F., American Academy of Pediatric, American Heart Association Subcommittee on Pediatric Resuscitation. (1998). *Pediatric Advanced Life Support*. American Heart Association. Dallas, Texas. American Heart Association.
Curley, M. A. Q. (1998). Patient-Nurse Synergy: Optimizing Patients' Outcomes. *American Journal of Critical Care* 7(1): 64–72.
Kaplow, R. (2003). AACN Synergy Model for Patient Care: A Framework to Optimize Outcomes. *Critical Care Nurse* 23(Suppl. 1): 27–30.

10. Answer d

The symptoms described are consistent with laryngotracheobronchitis (croup). Epiglottitis is often manifested by muffled voice and weak cough. Bronchiolitis is characterized by increased mucus production, airway edema, small airway obstruction, and air trapping. A typical history includes 2 to 5 days of upper airway infection and fever, followed by development of tachypnea, wheezing, crackles, and retractions. Bacterial pneumonia is often characterized by high fever and sudden onset or may follow viral illness. Possible signs of infection include fever, cough, tachypnea, nasal flaring, cyanosis, crackles, change in behavior, and gastrointestinal symptoms such as anorexia, vomiting, diarrhea, and abdominal pain.

In this situation, the child is demonstrating high levels of vulnerability and low levels of stability. The child is highly susceptible and fragile, and is labile with a potential for compromised respiratory status. The nurse is exhibiting moderate levels of clinical judgment by collecting and interpreting complex patient data.

REFERENCES

Curley, M. A. Q. (1998). Patient-Nurse Synergy: Optimizing Patients' Outcomes. *American Journal of Critical Care* 7(1): 64–72.

Hazinski, M. F. (1999). *Manual of Pediatric Critical Care* (pp. 340–344). St. Louis, MO: Mosby, Inc.

Kaplow, R. (2003). AACN Synergy Model for Patient Care: A Framework to Optimize Outcomes. *Critical Care Nurse* 23(Suppl. 1): 27–30.

11. Answer d

Combining psychomotor skills with verbal instructions promotes adult learning principles and will assist the nurse in learning retention. This response provides for patient safety and promotes a learning environment. The response should not be negative in nature (i.e., patient reassignment or orientation record note).

The patient is exhibiting a high level of vulnerability due to the head injury and is minimally stable as demonstrated by the frequent ICP spikes.

The preceptor is demonstrating moderate levels as a facilitator of learning by responding in a manner that provides the orientee with a learning opportunity regarding care of the patient with increased ICP. The preceptor is exhibiting a high level of clinical judgment by quickly making a clinical decision based on observation of the patient's response to their environment and past experiential knowledge.

The orientee is demonstrating low levels of clinical inquiry by not responding to the ICP spikes based on the individual patient's condition and their response to the environment.

REFERENCES

Curley, M. A. Q. (1998). Patient-Nurse Synergy: Optimizing Patients' Outcomes. *American Journal of Critical Care* 7(1): 64–72.

Kaplow, R. (2003). AACN Synergy Model for Patient Care: A Framework to Optimize Outcomes. *Critical Care Nurse* 23(Suppl. 1): 27–30.

12. Answer c

Due to the language barriers in this situation, it is critical to have a basic understanding of the parents' knowledge of the current clinical condition of their child and what their expectations are before discussing a plan of care. Providing language appropriate literature or translator alone does not provide the family or PICU team with adequate information to develop a plan that meets the needs of the family or child.

The patient and family are exhibiting high levels of vulnerability because of the severity of the infant's clinical situation. The family is exhibiting low levels of ability to participate in decision making because of the language and cultural barriers present.

The nurse is exhibiting moderate levels of advocacy/moral agency by obtaining information regarding the parents' values to incorporate into the decision-making process. The nurse is exhibiting moderate levels of caring practices by being responsive to the uniqueness of the patient and family in this situation.

REFERENCES

Curley, M. A. Q. (1998). Patient-Nurse Synergy: Optimizing Patients' Outcomes. *American Journal of Critical Care* 7(1): 64–72.

Kaplow, R. (2003). AACN Synergy Model for Patient Care: A Framework to Optimize Outcomes. *Critical Care Nurse* 23(Suppl. 1): 27–30.

13. Answer a

Before a decision can be made regarding how best to handle the mother's apparent lack of knowledge, an assessment of her overall level of knowledge must be made. When this is done, a referral can be made to the appropriate source.

The patient and mother are exhibiting high levels of complexity because of the long-term care required after heart transplant. The mother is exhibiting low levels of ability to participate in the infant's care because of possible lack of knowledge or misunderstanding of the care.

The nurse is exhibiting moderate levels of facilitator of learning by understanding where the learner is before teaching can be effective. The nurse is exhibiting a high level of clinical judgment because cessation of immunosuppressive medications could be fatal for this infant.

REFERENCES

Curley, M. A. Q. (1998). Patient-Nurse Synergy: Optimizing Patients' Outcomes. *American Journal of Critical Care* 7(1): 64–72.

Kaplow, R. (2003). AACN Synergy Model for Patient Care: A Framework to Optimize Outcomes. *Critical Care Nurse* 23(Suppl. 1): 27–30.

14. Answer b

By introducing the research process through in-service meetings, the committee nurses ensure that the project has a greater chance of being successful by enlisting staff support. In addition, the potential for expanding the research process in the unit is greater.

The committee nurses are exhibiting a high level of clinical inquiry because of their desire to incorporate research into their clinical practice. They are exhibiting a high level of facilitator of learning by recognizing that the success of the research process depends on educating the nursing staff to enlist their support.

REFERENCES

Curley, M. A. Q. (1998). Patient-Nurse Synergy: Optimizing Patients' Outcomes. *American Journal of Critical Care* 7(1): 64–72.
Kaplow, R. (2003). AACN Synergy Model for Patient Care: A Framework to Optimize Outcomes. *Critical Care Nurse* 23(Suppl. 1): 27–30.

15. Answer c

By acknowledging the parents' right to have their beliefs, the nurse validates their values. By explaining the emergent need, the nurse demonstrates advocacy for the patient.

The patient is exhibiting a low level of stability because of the ongoing blood loss. The family is exhibiting a high level of participation in decision making in their insistence that they do not want the blood transfusion.

The nurse is exhibiting a moderate level of response to diversity by acknowledging the parents' beliefs. The nurse is exhibiting a high level of advocacy/moral agency by supporting the patient's right to receive the transfusion and spending time to explain the need to the family even though they were not supportive.

REFERENCES

Curley, M. A. Q. (1998). Patient-Nurse Synergy: Optimizing Patients' Outcomes. *American Journal of Critical Care* 7(1): 64–72.
Kaplow, R. (2003). AACN Synergy Model for Patient Care: A Framework to Optimize Outcomes. *Critical Care Nurse* 23(Suppl. 1): 27–30.

16. Answer b

Before making plans to resolve the problem (i.e., mandatory in-service meetings or competency review changes), the specific concerns must be identified. By meeting with the cardiologist, the nurses can ask specific questions to get at the real issue.

The nurses are showing a high level of collaboration by meeting directly with the cardiologist to address the concerns before making a plan to solve the problem.

REFERENCES

Curley, M. A. Q. (1998). Patient-Nurse Synergy: Optimizing Patients' Outcomes. *American Journal of Critical Care* 7(1): 64–72.

Kaplow, R. (2003). AACN Synergy Model for Patient Care: A Framework to Optimize Outcomes. *Critical Care Nurse* 23(Suppl. 1): 27–30.

17. Answer c

Although the other choices may well be part of the process, the best initial action would be to gather a group of those people who will be most closely involved in working with the monitors after they are selected.

The nurses are exhibiting a high level of collaboration by including all the different personnel who would be affected by the purchase of a monitoring system. They are exhibiting a moderate level of clinical inquiry by looking to utilize all resources to identify the best monitoring system for their needs.

REFERENCES

Curley, M. A. Q. (1998). Patient-Nurse Synergy: Optimizing Patients' Outcomes. *American Journal of Critical Care* 7(1): 64–72.

Kaplow, R. (2003). AACN Synergy Model for Patient Care: A Framework to Optimize Outcomes. *Critical Care Nurse* 23(Suppl. 1): 27–30.

18. Answer d

The nurse has an important role in helping families understand what is happening to their child. By directly speaking with the family regarding this child's behavior, he is helping the family cope with what has happened so they can develop an understanding of how they can participate in care.

The patient is exhibiting a high level of complexity related to the severity of the brain injury sustained and the inability of the family to fully understand what it means. The patient is exhibiting a low level of resiliency related to poor ability to bounce back quickly from this insult.

The nurse is exhibiting a high level of facilitator of learning by taking the time and initiative to help the parents understand what they are seeing and why. The nurse is exhibiting a moderate level of clinical judgment by providing the family with accurate information regarding the pathology behind the exhibited behaviors of the child.

REFERENCES

Curley, M. A. Q. (1998). Patient-Nurse Synergy: Optimizing Patients' Outcomes. *American Journal of Critical Care* 7(1): 64–72.

Kaplow, R. (2003). AACN Synergy Model for Patient Care: A Framework to Optimize Outcomes. *Critical Care Nurse* 23(Suppl. 1): 27–30.

19. Answer c

The patient is hypotensive, tachycardic, and has poor perfusion with fluid losses related to hyperglycemia through the urine output. The patient is exhibiting low levels of stability.

The nurse is exhibiting moderate levels of clinical judgment in understanding the clinical signs and symptoms of hypovolemia.

REFERENCES

Curley, M. A. Q. (1998). Patient-Nurse Synergy: Optimizing Patients' Outcomes. *American Journal of Critical Care* 7(1): 64–72.

Kaplow, R. (2003). AACN Synergy Model for Patient Care: A Framework to Optimize Outcomes. *Critical Care Nurse* 23(Suppl. 1): 27–30.

20. Answer a

Patients with DKA can be significantly dehydrated due to osmotic diuresis from hyperglycemia. The patient has a low BP, is tachycardic, and has poor peripheral perfusion. Initially, fluid resuscitation should be aggressive but the entire deficit should not be too rapid because of the risk of electrolyte imbalance and fluid shifts resulting in cerebral edema. The patient is showing low levels of stability because of the hypovolemic shock being exhibited.

The nurse is showing high levels of clinical judgment because of the need to have a good understanding of the underlying pathophysiology of diabetic ketoacidosis to make the right fluid resuscitation decisions.

REFERENCES

Curley, M. A. Q. (1998). Patient-Nurse Synergy: Optimizing Patients' Outcomes. *American Journal of Critical Care* 7(1): 64–72.

Kaplow, R. (2003). AACN Synergy Model for Patient Care: A Framework to Optimize Outcomes. *Critical Care Nurse* 23(Suppl. 1): 27–30.

21. Answer c

Patients with DKA and very elevated glucose levels have intracellular hypoglycemia and hypokalemia. As glucose levels return to normal, it is important to add glucose and potassium to the IV fluids to prevent overcorrection with resulting hypoglycemia that can contribute to the development of cerebral edema and hypokalemia.

The patient is exhibiting moderate levels of resiliency by showing good improvement with therapy. The patient is showing moderate levels of predictability as demonstrated by expected improvement in labs and vital signs.

The nurse is showing moderate levels of clinical judgment by understanding the underlying pathophysiology related to management of DKA and applying that to the specific fluid needs of this patient at this time.

REFERENCES

Curley, M. A. Q. (1998). Patient-Nurse Synergy: Optimizing Patients' Outcomes. *American Journal of Critical Care* 7(1): 64–72.

Kaplow, R. (2003). AACN Synergy Model for Patient Care: A Framework to Optimize Outcomes. *Critical Care Nurse* 23(Suppl. 1): 27–30.

22. Answer a

This family fears that they will not be able to perform the care so that they will ultimately be able to take their baby home. It is important to allow the family time to get used to the things they will need to be taught and gradually have them start taking over. Providing the family with information too soon will just overwhelm them further and increase their fears.

The patient is exhibiting high levels of complexity related to the significant technology required. The family is exhibiting low levels of resource availability because they are so frightened they can't take the information in to be able to start learning and managing the care.

The nurse is exhibiting high levels of caring practices and facilitator of learning by understanding that she must work with the family slowly and allow them to develop confidence in their abilities.

REFERENCES

Curley, M. A. Q. (1998). Patient-Nurse Synergy: Optimizing Patients' Outcomes. *American Journal of Critical Care* 7(1): 64–72.

Kaplow, R. (2003). AACN Synergy Model for Patient Care: A Framework to Optimize Outcomes. *Critical Care Nurse* 23(Suppl. 1): 27–30.

23. Answer c

The hypotension, tachycardia, hypoxemia, and delayed capillary refill time indicate poor perfusion and the gallop rhythm and crackles demonstrate myocardial dysfunction all pointing toward cardiogenic shock. The patient is demonstrating high levels of complexity related to the history and presentation.

The nurse is demonstrating moderate levels of clinical judgment by being able to apply the physical exam findings to a pathophysiology.

REFERENCES

Curley, M. A. Q. (1998). Patient-Nurse Synergy: Optimizing Patients' Outcomes. *American Journal of Critical Care* 7(1): 64–72.

Kaplow, R. (2003). AACN Synergy Model for Patient Care: A Framework to Optimize Outcomes. *Critical Care Nurse* 23(Suppl. 1): 27–30.

24. Answer c

This patient is demonstrating signs of cardiogenic shock probably due to a viral myocarditis. It would be important to improve cardiac output by improving myocardial function and decreasing systemic vascular resistance. Choice a might be true for the steroids but not initially. Choice b—with severe myocardial dysfunction and anticoagulation—is important but again not initially. Choice d, inotropic support, is very important but fluid resuscitation could be detrimental given the results of the physical exam.

The patient is exhibiting minimal levels of stability as demonstrated by the vital signs and of resiliency as demonstrated by the physical exam. The nurse is exhibiting high levels of clinical judgment by assessing the patient, utilizing knowledge of pathophysiology, and developing a plan of care to manage the problem.

REFERENCES

Curley, M. A. Q. (1998). Patient-Nurse Synergy: Optimizing Patients' Outcomes. *American Journal of Critical Care* 7(1): 64–72.

Kaplow, R. (2003). AACN Synergy Model for Patient Care: A Framework to Optimize Outcomes. *Critical Care Nurse* 23(Suppl. 1): 27–30.

25. Answer b

Although each of the responses is important, maintaining ongoing adequate sedation will help prevent the initial pulmonary artery spikes that can spiral downward to hypoxemia and hypercarbia that can then result in a potentially fatal pulmonary hypertensive crisis.

The patient is exhibiting minimal levels of stability as demonstrated by the elevated PA pressures with movement. The patient is exhibiting minimal levels of resiliency as demonstrated by the inability to maintain a hemodynamic steady state with minimal stimulation.

REFERENCES

Curley, M. A. Q. (1998). Patient-Nurse Synergy: Optimizing Patients' Outcomes. *American Journal of Critical Care* 7(1): 64–72.

Kaplow, R. (2003). AACN Synergy Model for Patient Care: A Framework to Optimize Outcomes. *Critical Care Nurse* 23(Suppl. 1): 27–30.

CHAPTER 20

THE ACUTELY AND CRITICALLY ILL NEONATAL PATIENT SAMPLE QUESTIONS

Beth C. Diehl-Svrjcek, MS, RN, CCRN, CCM, NNP, LNCC

INTRODUCTION

The following questions have been developed to provide examples of questions that integrate the patient and nurse characteristics of the AACN Synergy Model. The scenarios and questions in this chapter focus on acutely and critically ill neonatal patients in a variety of patient care settings. Each question is followed by four choices. One answer is the best answer. An annotated key at the end of the questions provides the correct choice along with a rationale for why the other choices are not the best, based on the AACN Synergy Model.

1. The mother of an extremely premature neonate expresses anxiety when the nurse suggests that she can lightly stroke her baby during visits. To ease the mother's anxiety, the nurse should initially:
   a. Give the mother a pamphlet about maternal-infant bonding.
   b. Explore the basis of the mother's anxiety.
   c. Demonstrate proper stroking technique to the mother.
   d. Refer the mother to a social worker for support.

2. Parents of a neonate who has been diagnosed with Trisomy 13 tell the nurse during a bedside visit that they want the baby resuscitated in the event of cardiorespiratory arrest. The nurse should best assist these parents by:
   a. Requesting that they speak with the neonatal intensive care unit (NICU) social worker.
   b. Referring them to a support group for neonates with Trisomy 13
   c. Scheduling an interdisciplinary meeting with parents and the NICU team.
   d. Referring them to appropriate clergy for support.

3. During the NICU orientation process, a nurse is assigned to care for a neonate who is immediately status post VP shunt placement. The preceptor observes the orientee positioning the head of the neonate so that they are lying directly on the shunt. The preceptor should best correct this improper positioning of the neonate by:
   a. Repositioning the head of the neonate immediately.
   b. Explaining to the orientee principles of postop care.
   c. Directing the orientee to reposition the head of the neonate.
   d. Reporting the orientee's actions to the nurse manager.

4. A preterm neonate has pathological jaundice that will require exchange transfusion per bilirubin level. The parents are Jehovah's Witnesses and oppose the administration of blood products. The attending physician has informed the parents that a court order will be pursued so that the exchange can be completed. The parents express anger toward the NICU staff. The NICU nurse should best support these parents by:
   a. Notifying the hospital administration of the situation.
   b. Referring them to the NICU social worker for counseling.
   c. Initiating a call to the hospital clergy for spiritual support.
   d. Validating the parents' religious beliefs regarding blood transfusions.

5. A community hospital has received funding to upgrade from a Level I NICU to a Level III NICU. An interdisciplinary task force has been appointed by hospital administration to oversee the project. The proposed physical layout of the NICU does not promote neonatal developmentally appropriate care related to lighting and noise issues. The NICU nurse appointed to the task force should take which of the following actions to address this situation:
   a. Present studies regarding the importance of a developmentally focused NICU environment.
   b. Develop strategies to negate the effects of the light and noise stimuli in the current model.
   c. Report the deficits of the current physical model to the nursing administration.
   d. Speak with the neonatology director to garner support for a change to the physical layout.

6. A new suctioning protocol to decrease tracheal trauma has been developed by a NICU clinical practice committee per evidenced-based research. For the protocol to be successfully implemented by all nursing staff, the nurse liaison to this committee should:
   a. Distribute copies of the protocol to each nursing staff member.
   b. Work with the nurse manager to assure compliance to the protocol.
   c. Provide information during staff meetings that supports research basis.
   d. Provide implementation summary to committee 18 months later.

7. The mother who utilized heroin throughout her pregnancy expresses the desire to provide breast milk for her premature neonate. To properly address this situation, the NICU nurse should:
   a. Refer the mother to the hospital-based lactation consultant.
   b. Secure an electric breast pump for the mother to utilize.
   c. Review the process for collection of breast milk with the mother.
   d. Review the protocol for breast milk usage with drug-exposed neonates.

8. A 14-year-old mother comes to the NICU with her mother to visit her recently admitted premature infant. The infant's grandmother monopolizes the conversation with the bedside nurse stating her daughter is "too young" to understand the baby's medical problems and needs. To promote bonding between this teenage mom and her neonate, the nurse should:
   a. Refer the family to the NICU social worker for counseling.
   b. Disregard the grandmother's comments about her daughter's capabilities.
   c. Encourage the mother to touch and stroke the infant during NICU visits.
   d. Refer the family to the adolescent clinic for post-NICU primary care.

9. A Level III NICU is establishing a protocol for back/convalescent transports to lower level nurseries across the state. The NICU nurse serving on this committee is responsible for researching the clinical nursing capabilities of the outlying facilities. Which of the following initial actions by the NICU nurse should make this process most successful?
   a. Speaking with the physician administrator from each facility.
   b. Sending a clinical questionnaire to the nursery nurse manager.
   c. Personally visiting the nursery of each facility.
   d. Querying pediatricians with facility-specific admitting privileges.

10. A new type of intravenous catheter is being piloted for possible purchase by the nursing staff of a NICU. The manufacturer cites clinical research that the flexibility of this particular catheter decreases the rate of intravenous infiltration. However, the nursing staff documents a higher rate of IV infiltration during the pilot phase. The NICU nurse coordinating this pilot should:
    a. Return the remaining IV catheters to the manufacturer.
    b. Consult the neonatologist for further direction.
    c. Contact the company's clinical representative.
    d. Discuss the issue at the next nursing staff meeting.

11. The mother of a 30-week neonate is pleased when she witnesses her baby sucking on a pacifier while in the isolette. She asks the nurse if she can now feed her baby with a bottle because the baby is sucking on the pacifier so well. To educate the mother in safe feeding practices, the NICU nurse should:
    a. Explain the need for suck/swallow coordination with nipple feeding.
    b. Encourage the mother to attend well-baby care class.
    c. Provide the mother with written materials about non-nutritive sucking.
    d. Discuss the issue with the mother at the next bedside visit.

12. A lesbian couple has a premature neonate admitted to the NICU. They visit the neonate daily and are openly affectionate to each other at the bedside. These behaviors are offensive to family members visiting other neonates. The other families request that the baby be moved to a separate room within the NICU. The NICU nurse should best resolve this situation by:
    a. Addressing the affectionate behavior with the couple directly.
    b. Placing a privacy screen near the bedside when the couple visits.
    c. Referring the couple to the NICU social worker.
    d. Scheduling a team meeting of NICU staff.

13. A Level III NICU facility has received a grant to fund an extra corporeal membrane oxygenation (ECMO) program. The committee has been working to coordinate the training for the program. Contrary to the committee's recommendation, the physician committee chairperson does not see the need for competency-based training. The NICU nurse serving on this committee should take which of the following actions to promote a competency-based training approach for nursing staff providing bedside care during ECMO therapy:
    a. Present studies regarding the effectiveness of competency-based training.
    b. Discuss the concept with the other committee members privately.
    c. Report the proposed training to the NICU nurse manager.
    d. Explore the training programs of other existing ECMO centers.

14. A neonate is admitted to the NICU with a diagnosis of ambiguous genitalia. The parents are clearly stressed by this diagnosis during their first bedside visit. The mother expresses guilt for cigarette smoking during her pregnancy indicating "I know I caused this problem with my smoking." The nurse should:
    a. Refer the parents to the neonatologist for an explanation.
    b. Offer a counseling session with the NICU social worker.
    c. Explain the anatomic basis for ambiguous genitalia formation.
    d. Offer information regarding a local support group.

15. The neonate of a mother with a history of heroin abuse is admitted to the NICU for respiratory distress. On day three of the neonate's life, the mother asks the bedside nurse during her visit why the baby is so "fussy and shaky." When the nurse explains that these behaviors are symptoms of neonatal drug withdrawal, the mother becomes upset, stating she "never took no drugs" during her pregnancy. The mother and baby both tested positive for opiates in urine samples. The NICU nurse should:
    a. Allow the mother to express her emotions.
    b. Contact the hospital substance abuse counselor.
    c. Ask security staff to escort the mother from the unit.
    d. Ask the neonatologist to speak with the mother.

16. A neonate, prenatally diagnosed with anencephaly, is admitted to the NICU immediately after delivery. A plan of compassionate care is implemented. The father does not want the mother to see the baby at any point, stating that it would be "too devastating" for her. The NICU nurse should:
    a. Give the father his own picture of the baby.
    b. Contact hospital clergy for parental support.
    c. Tell the father that request cannot be honored.
    d. Agree with the father regarding maternal visitation.

17. The NICU team is developing a protocol for ventilation with nitric oxide (NO) as an available therapy for neonates with Primary Pulmonary Hypertension of the Newborn (PPHN). It is a multidisciplinary effort and involves the medical staff, respiratory therapy (RT), and nursing staff. However, hospital administration is hesitant to provide funding for this equipment, given projected costs and the number of neonates that may be eligible for this therapy on an annual basis. The NICU nurse, in concert with the medical staff, should take which of the following initial actions:
    a. Perform a retrospective chart review to determine past eligible NO candidates.
    b. Ask the NO contract representative to speak with hospital administration.
    c. Present studies regarding standard of care for neonates with PPHN.
    d. Speak with the nurse manager to request a budget reallocation.

18. A nurse orientee is caring for a 24-week neonate receiving surfactant replacement therapy immediately following delivery room resuscitation. The preceptor notices that the orientee is preparing to suction the airway shortly after the surfactant administration has been completed due to suspected airway obstruction. The preceptor should initially:
    a. Allow the orientee to complete the suctioning procedure.
    b. Instruct the orientee to summon RT for assistance.
    c. Explain the action of exogenous surfactant on pulmonary system.
    d. Assist the orientee to reposition the neonate's endotracheal tube.

19. A nurse caring for a 6-day-old premature neonate notices a recent increase in apneic and bradycardic episodes combined with lethargy and temperature instability. The stool present in the diaper tests guaiac positive. To properly address this situation, the nurse should:
    a. Place the neonate in a double-walled isolette.
    b. Notify the physician of these clinical findings.
    c. Continue bolus enteral feedings as ordered.
    d. Suggest the administration of a loading dose of caffeine.

20. A pediatric resident is preparing to re-insert an obstructed chest tube in a neonate. The NICU nurse requests that the neonate be medicated for pain prior to the procedure. The resident declines to write the order for an analgesic, stating there is limited time to complete the procedure before rounds begin so the work must proceed. The NICU nurse should:
    a. Institute nonpharmacological pain control measures such as nonnutritive sucking.

    b. Notify the attending neonatologist to obtain an order for analgesia.

    c. Utilize the Premature Infant Pain Profile to assess the pain score during the procedure.

    d. Report the incident to the chief pediatric resident.

21. A neonate status post repair of tracheal-esophageal fistula (TEF) is having difficulty with oral feedings. The neonate has been dependent on partial gastrostomy feedings and has had intermittent episodes of vomiting. The parents are expressing high levels of frustration and the occupational therapist disagrees with the neonatologist on the overall feeding plan. The NICU nurse should best address the situation by:

    a. Referring the parents to a NICU parent support group.

    b. Asking the neonatologist to speak with the parents directly.

    c. Scheduling a team meeting to discuss the feeding plan.

    d. Contacting the supervisor of the occupational therapist.

22. A neonate is born with Hypoplastic Left Heart Syndrome (HLHS) along with multiple congenital anomalies. After thorough discussion with the NICU team, the parents decline surgical intervention or cardiac transplantation and elect the compassionate care treatment option until death occurs. The maternal grandparents highly oppose this decision and express anger toward the parents during bedside visits. The nurse should best assist the parents by:

    a. Referring the family to the NICU social worker for counseling.

    b. Restricting the grandparents from bedside visitation.

    c. Reviewing the treatment options for HLHS with the grandparents.

    d. Requesting a review of the case by the hospital ethics committee.

23. A study involving extremely low birth weight neonates is being planned in a Level III NICU by the clinical practice committee to evaluate differing methods of skin care among the nursing staff. One group of neonates will be treated with a water miscible ointment; the other group will serve as the nontreated control group. For the study to be successfully completed, the nurse coordinating this study should:

    a. Hold all results regarding the study until it is completely finished.

    b. Periodically inform the nursing staff of the study status, i.e., enrollment numbers.

    c. Inform the nurse manager of any instances of noncompliance with the study protocol.

    d. Seek family involvement to encourage the study enrollment.

24. A term neonate is admitted to the NICU following respiratory distress in the delivery room. The neonate has no signs of respiratory distress when crying but becomes cyanotic at rest. The nurse is unable to pass a catheter through either nare during the admitting assessment. The nurse should suspect which disease state and ready which piece of equipment:

    a. Pierre Robin Syndrome, Breck nipple.

    b. Choanal Atresia, oral airway.

c. Vascular Ring, nasal airway.
d. Laryngotracheal Cleft, ET tube.

25. A mother is visiting her ex-23-week neonate who is to undergo laser surgery in both eyes related to retinopathy of prematurity (ROP) at threshold. The mother has spoken with the pediatric ophthalmologist and consented to the procedure but expresses anxiety that her baby may be blind despite the interventions. To ease the mother's anxiety, the nurse should:
a. Refer the mother to the local school for the blind for resources.
b. Request that the neonatologist speak to the mother regarding the procedure.
c. Refer the mother to the pediatric ophthalmologist for a specific prognosis.
d. Explore with the mother her knowledge base regarding ROP/laser surgery.

ANSWER KEY AND RATIONALES TO ACUTELY AND CRITICALLY ILL NEONATAL PATIENT SAMPLE QUESTIONS

1. Answer b

By exploring the mother's anxiety, the nurse can determine the basis for the anxiety and incorporate measures into the plan of care to facilitate ongoing bonding activities. A pamphlet about bonding, a social work referral, and demonstration of stroking techniques would be secondary interventions, not initial interventions.

REFERENCE

Kenner, C., & Amlung, S. (1999). Families in Crisis. In J. Deacon and P. O'Neill, eds. *Core Curriculum for Neonatal Intensive Care Nursing* (p. 646). Philadelphia: W.B. Saunders.

2. Answer c

Because Trisomy 13 is incompatible with life, resuscitation would be futile treatment. A meeting with all members of the NICU team would best address the medical and ethical concerns in this situation. A referral to clergy and/or social work in isolation would not deal with the futility of care issue. The nurse is demonstrating moral agency in this scenario.

REFERENCE

Schiefelbein, J. (1999). Genetics and Fetal Anomalies. In J. Deacon and P. O'Neill, eds. *Core Curriculum for Neonatal Intensive Care Nursing* (p. 557). Philadelphia: W.B. Saunders.

3. Answer c

Retention of learning for the orientee is higher when psychomotor skills are combined with verbal instructions. This action would provide for patient safety and foster adult learning principles and should not be punitive in nature, i.e., report to the nurse manager. The nurse is demonstrating the characteristic of facilitator of learning.

REFERENCE

Paige, P., & Carney, P. (2002). Neurologic Disorders. In G. B. Merenstein & S. L. Gardner, eds. *Handbook of Neonatal Intensive Care* (p. 649). St. Louis, MO: Mosby.

4. Answer d

The parents' beliefs will not be altered by any of the other interventions listed. Only by recognizing and appreciating their religious beliefs regarding blood transfusions will the parents be able to maintain open communication with the NICU nurse and other team members. This nurse is demonstrating the characteristic of response to diversity.

REFERENCE

Verklan, M. T. (1999). Legal Issues in the NICU. In J. Deacon & P. O'Neill, eds. *Core Curriculum for Neonatal Intensive Care Nursing* (p. 768). Philadelphia: W.B. Saunders.

5. Answer a

The task force may be unaware of the importance of the NICU environment on developmental care and may be utilizing other criteria in determining the layout, i.e., physical space, cost, and staffing issues. By presenting studies to this interdisciplinary group validating the need for alterations to the physical layout, the task force can collaborate to take all logistical, cost, and clinical issues into consideration. The nurse is demonstrating the characteristic of collaboration.

REFERENCE

Koch, S. (1999). Developmental Support in the Neonatal Intensive Care Unit. In J. Deacon & P. O'Neill, eds. *Core Curriculum for Neonatal Intensive Care Nursing* (pp. 522–526). Philadelphia: W.B. Saunders.

6. Answer c

Changes in clinical practice must be supported by research and staff knowledge of that research as per adult learning theory for change to be most effective.

Simply distributing the protocol as a stand-alone venture exclusive of staff meetings may not be as effective. The nurse is demonstrating the characteristic of clinical inquiry.

REFERENCE

Cornell, W. (1999). Research. In J. Deacon & P. O'Neill, eds. *Core Curriculum for Neonatal Intensive Care Nursing* (pp. 732–740). Philadelphia: W.B. Saunders.

7. Answer d

The primary concern is to determine if the breast milk contains drug metabolites that would be unsafe for the infant to consume. The first step would be to review hospital protocol to determine the next course of action, which may include any of the other choices. The nurse is demonstrating the characteristic of clinical judgment.

REFERENCE

Botham, S. (1999). Perinatal Substance Abuse. In J. Deacon & P. O'Neill, eds. *Core Curriculum for Neonatal Intensive Care Nursing* (p. 630). Philadelphia: W.B. Saunders.

8. Answer c

Engaging the mother during visits to the NICU, as a demonstration of her abilities to the grandmother, is essential to promote bonding with her neonate. Although social work interventions and an adolescent clinic follow-up would be helpful, bedside interventions are most important. The nurse is demonstrating the characteristic of response to diversity.

REFERENCE

Kenner, C., & Amlung, S. (1999). Families in Crisis. In J. Deacon & P. O'Neill, eds. *Core Curriculum for Neonatal Intensive Care Nursing* (pp. 646–647). Philadelphia: W.B. Saunders.

9. Answer c

Because the NICU nurse is most concerned about the nursing capabilities, the nurse manager would be able to provide information on staffing, knowledge level of staff, status of policies and procedures on neonatal care, and so forth. A site visit may be appropriate but not as an initial intervention. It is unlikely the physicians would have this nursing-based information. The nurse is demonstrating the characteristic of system thinking.

REFERENCE

Bowen, S. L. (1999). Neonatal Transport. In J. Deacon & P. O'Neill, eds. *Core Curriculum for Neonatal Intensive Care Nursing* (p. 705). Philadelphia: W.B. Saunders.

10. Answer c

The clinical representative should be contacted to quickly meet with the NICU staff and review the issues surrounding the increased rate of infiltrations. Termination of the pilot would be inappropriate until equipment failure versus staff insertion technique is ruled out. Because infiltration as a clinical issue has been identified, it must be dealt with prior to the next scheduled staff meeting. The nurse is demonstrating the characteristic of clinical inquiry.

REFERENCE

Cornell, W. (1999). Research. In J. Deacon & P. O'Neill, eds. *Core Curriculum for Neonatal Intensive Care Nursing* (pp. 734–740). Philadelphia: W.B. Saunders.

11. Answer a

Because safe nipple feedings cannot be initiated until 33–34 weeks post conceptual age for neurological maturity reasons, the mother requires immediate education on this issue. Although information about well-baby care and non-nutritive sucking may be helpful, it will not fulfill her most pressing educational need. The nurse is demonstrating the characteristic of facilitator of learning.

REFERENCE

Koch, S. (1999). Developmental Support in the Neonatal Intensive Care Unit. In J. Deacon & P. O'Neill, eds. *Core Curriculum for Neonatal Intensive Care Nursing* (p. 530). Philadelphia: W.B. Saunders.

12. Answer d

A successful solution will involve discussion among several members of the NICU team to explore appropriate alternatives to deal effectively with the visitation issue. Although a privacy screen and social work support is feasible, it does establish a universal team approach that is essential to address the diversity issue. The nurse is demonstrating the nurse characteristic of response to diversity.

REFERENCE

Kenner, C., & Amlung, S. (1999). Families in Crisis. In J. Deacon and P. O'Neill, eds. *Core Curriculum for Neonatal Intensive Care Nursing* (pp. 640–642). Philadelphia: W.B. Saunders.

13. Answer a

The chairperson may be unaware of the importance of competency-based training for providing care to a neonate receiving ECMO. By presenting studies validating the need for this type of training, the chairperson may be more likely to side with the other committee members and agree to this approach. It may be helpful to query other centers but a literature search will be most effective. The nurse is demonstrating the characteristic of collaboration.

REFERENCE

Lund, C. H. (1999). Extracorporeal Membrane Oxygenation in the Neonate. In J. Deacon & P. O'Neill, eds. *Core Curriculum for Neonatal Intensive Care Nursing* (pp. 192–200). Philadelphia: W.B. Saunders.

14. Answer c

The parents must first understand that ambiguous genitalia is the result of a defect in embryological development and is not caused by an external factor such as smoking. Although they may ultimately speak with the neonatologist and social worker, an initial discussion regarding the facts about their baby's diagnosis will allay their guilt. The nurse is demonstrating the characteristic of facilitator of learning.

REFERENCE

Kenner, C., and Amlung, S. (1999). Families in Crisis. In J. Deacon and P. O'Neill, eds. *Core Curriculum for Neonatal Intensive Care Nursing* (pp. 647–648). Philadelphia: W.B. Saunders.

15. Answer a

The mother must first express her feelings before she can move further to address her drug abuse issues and seek help for herself as well as her baby. She need not be removed by security from the unit unless her behaviors threaten others in the NICU. The substance abuse counselor would be the next step in the process but not an initial intervention. The nurse is demonstrating the characteristic of caring practices.

REFERENCE

Botham, S. (1999). Perinatal Substance Abuse. In J. Deacon & P. O'Neill, eds. *Core Curriculum for Neonatal Intensive Care Nursing* (pp. 631–633). Philadelphia: W.B. Saunders.

16. Answer c

One parent cannot limit the other parent's visitation rights unless court ordered. Because it is likely this baby will have a relatively short life span, it is important that the mother be allowed to visit if that is indeed her desire. A picture should be taken for both parents to have for future viewing. The nurse is demonstrating the characteristic of advocacy.

REFERENCE

MuCulloch, M. (1999). Neurologic Disorders. In J. Deacon & P. O'Neill, eds. *Core Curriculum for Neonatal Intensive Care Nursing* (p. 480). Philadelphia: W.B. Saunders.

17. Answer c

It would be most important to focus on current treatment protocols within the discipline of neonatology to support the equipment acquisition. Data from a retro chart review could also demonstrate need as a secondary intervention. The nurse is demonstrating the characteristic of systems thinking.

REFERENCE

Hagedorn, M. E., Gardner, S., & Abman, S. (2002). Respiratory Diseases. In G. B. Merenstein and S. L. Gardner, eds. *Handbook of Neonatal Intensive Care* (pp. 548–50). St. Louis, MO: Mosby.

18. Answer b

Airway obstruction may occur during surfactant administration because of the viscosity of the secretions. An increase in mechanical support may be required until the surfactant is spread from the airways to the alveoli. Respiratory therapy would be able to provide this immediate care. Suctioning would serve to remove the surfactant from the pulmonary tree and would negate the desired effect as would repositioning of the ET tube. The nurse is demonstrating the characteristic of facilitator of learning.

REFERENCE

Gomella, T. L. (1999). *Neonatology: Management, Procedures, On-Call Problems, Diseases, and Drugs* 4th ed. (p. 58). New York, NY: The McGraw Hill Companies, Inc.

19. Answer b

The symptoms are nonspecific signs of suspected necrotizing enterocolitis (NEC). The physician must be notified immediately to prevent progression of the disease. Although these early signs may also be indicative of neonatal sepsis, feeds are stopped to allow for bowel rest. A caffeine bolus and utilization of a double-walled isolette are not effective treatments for NEC. The nurse is demonstrating the characteristic of clinical judgment.

REFERENCE

Gomella, T. L. (1999). *Neonatology: Management, Procedures, On-Call Problems, Diseases, and Drugs* 4th ed. (pp. 452–454). New York, NY: The McGraw Hill Companies, Inc.

20. Answer b

Research has demonstrated that neonates should have adequate pain management during invasive procedures. This procedure should not be initiated until pharmacological pain control measures have been instituted. Certainly, nonpharmacological measures and a pain assessment tool can be utilized but not without pharmacological intervention. The nurse is demonstrating the characteristic of caring practices.

REFERENCE

Bildner, J. (1999). Neonatal Pain Management. In J. Deacon & P. O'Neill, eds. *Core Curriculum for Neonatal Intensive Care Nursing* (pp. 512–513). Philadelphia: W.B. Saunders.

21. Answer c

A team meeting would be the optimal avenue to assess current feeding interventions and redefine the plan of care for all parties involved. Individual specific interventions would be ineffective. The nurse is demonstrating the characteristic of collaboration.

REFERENCE

Watson, R. L. (1999). Gastrointestinal Disorders. In J. Deacon & P. O'Neill, eds. *Core Curriculum for Neonatal Intensive Care Nursing* (pp. 263–265). Philadelphia: W.B. Saunders.

22. Answer a

Because the parents and NICU team have already determined the treatment decision, further explanations or review by the ethics committee for the grandparents would be inappropriate. Counseling by the social worker may assist this family to express their differing opinions within a therapeutic milieu and help the grandparents understand the parents' decision. The nurse is demonstrating the characteristic of advocacy/moral agency.

REFERENCE

Gomella, T. L. (1999). *Neonatology: Management, Procedures, On-Call Problems, Diseases and Drugs* 4th ed. (p. 339). New York, NY: The McGraw Hill Companies, Inc.

23. Answer b

Periodic updates will serve to maintain awareness of the nursing staff and interest in study protocol until a final summary can be provided to the staff. Family involvement is desirable but not required. The nurse is demonstrating the characteristic of clinical inquiry.

REFERENCE

Cornell, W. (1999). Research. In J. Deacon and P. O'Neill, eds. *Core Curriculum for Neonatal Intensive Care Nursing* (pp. 732–740). Philadelphia: W.B. Saunders.

24. Answer b

Choanal atresia is a congenital blockage of the posterior nares. Because neonates are obligatory nose breathers, they manifest respiratory distress at rest versus during crying episodes when the mouth is open so an oral airway will alleviate symptoms. Pierre Robin involves mandibular hypoplasia and prone positioning, vascular ring causes stridor. Laryngotracheal cleft is an incomplete separation of the larynx and esophagus and usually warrants surgical correction. The nurse is demonstrating the characteristic of clinical judgment.

REFERENCE

Gomella, T. L. (1999). *Neonatology: Management, Procedures, On-Call Problems, Diseases and Drugs* 4th ed. (pp. 536–537). New York, NY: The McGraw Hill Companies, Inc.

25. Answer d

Because the procedure has not yet been completed, the opthomologist may not be able to provide a specific prognosis. The mother's concerns would be best addressed by assessing her level of knowledge to determine what future interventions would be most helpful, i.e., educational materials and/or support group or community resources, pending the outcome of the surgery. The nurse is demonstrating the characteristic of caring practices.

REFERENCE

Hagedorn, M. E., Gardner, S., & Abman, S. (2002). Respiratory Diseases. In G. B. Merenstein & S. L. Gardner, eds. *Handbook of Neonatal Intensive Care* (pp. 525–530). St. Louis, MO: Mosby.

CHAPTER 21

ADVANCED PRACTICE SAMPLE QUESTIONS: ADULT NURSE PRACTITIONER

Darla Ura, MA, RN, APRN, BC
Linda L. Steele, PhD, RN, APRN, ANP-BC

INTRODUCTION

The following questions have been developed to provide examples of questions that integrate the patient and nurse practitioner (NP) characteristics of the AACN Synergy Model. The scenarios and questions in this chapter focus on the role of the NP in a variety of patient care settings. Each question is followed by four choices. One answer is the best answer. An annotated key at the end of the questions provides the correct choice along with a rationale for why the other choices are not the best, based on the AACN Synergy Model.

SCENARIO 1

Questions 1–4 refer to the following scenario.

A patient has returned from a four-vessel bypass and is in the ICU. Her past medical history is significant for uncontrolled noninsulin-dependent diabetes mellitus (NIDDM) for 14 years, hypertension for 10 years, and a family history of coronary artery disease.

1. The nurse reports that the patient has had 500 cc blood loss through the chest tube during the first 2 hours. Which of the following would be the highest priority?
   a. Administer two units of packed red blood cells immediately.
   b. Contact the patient's family and inform that their family member is in a crisis.
   c. Order a stat lab for platelets and coagulation profile (ACT, PT, or PTT).
   d. Notify the collaborating physician and prepare to return the patient to the operating room.

2. It is now 4 hours later and the patient has continued to drain blood at a rate of 150 to 200 cc per hour into the chest tube. Lab data are as follows:

PT	21.3 sec
PTT	37.4 sec
INR	1.4 sec
Hgb	9.2 Gm/dl
Hct	27.6%
Platelets	152×10^3

You, the nurse practitioner, are present and have followed protocol. The next line of intervention would be to:

a. Consult with the surgeon to possibly return the patient to the operating room.

b. Notify the family that the patient must go back to surgery.

c. Administer two units of fresh frozen plasma and 10 mg Vitamin K.

d. Order a repeat CBC and chemical profile.

3. The patient is now 1-week postop and is ambulatory. All tubes and wires have been removed. The patient has a blood sugar that remains in the low 200s and has been maintained with sliding scale insulin. The patient is now ready for discharge. Which of the following orders would be important for the NP to address?

a. Limit activity to no more than 10 minutes per day.

b. Monitor the pulse rate while being active to ensure that the heart rate does not go above 60.

c. Return to her general internal medicine provider as soon as possible to assist with her blood sugar regulation.

d. Increase her dose of oral hypoglycemic agents to four times a day.

4. It is now 5 years since the patient had bypass surgery. She reports to the NP that she is extremely short of breath and fatigued. It is determined that she is now in heart failure. Which of the following medication regimens would be the first line of treatment for this patient?

a. Calcium channel blockers, diuretics, and nitroglycerine.

b. Diuretics, beta blockers, and digoxin.

c. Digoxin, ACE inhibitors, and calcium blocker.

d. Diuretics and ACE inhibitors.

SCENARIO 2

Questions 5–8 refer to the following scenario.

A 70-year-old man presents to the ED complaining of sudden onset of severe abdominal pain with concomitant vomiting. His history is significant for one pack-per-day cigarette smoking, COPD, hypercholesterolemia, insulin dependent diabetes, atrial fibrillation, and congestive heart failure. He denies any past history of hypertension or renal problems. His vital signs show a temperature of

101°F, heart rate of 124, blood pressure of 90/40, and respirations of 24. His abdomen is mildly tender with no rigidity. He has had blood-tinged diarrhea since admission to the ED.

5. Which of the following lab tests should the NP order for this patient?
   a. CBC, chemistry panel, and arterial blood gas.
   b. CBC, chemistry panel, and haptoglobin.
   c. CBC, liver function tests, and ionized calcium.
   d. CBC, coagulation profile, and troponin.

6. The patient is diagnosed with acute mesenteric ischemia. The next interventions that NP will order should include:
   a. Ensure adequate ventilation and correct hypovolemia.
   b. Monitor vital signs and blood loss.
   c. Contact the patient's family and consult with an enterostomal therapist.
   d. Insert a nasogastric tube and monitor drainage.

7. With a confirmed diagnosis of acute mesenteric ischemia, the NP should anticipate that the next most important intervention would be to contact the:
   a. Family to come to the hospital.
   b. Surgeon for emergency bowel surgery.
   c. Chaplain to be with the patient.
   d. Blood bank for type and cross match.

8. The patient endures surgical intervention but has developed multiple organ dysfunction syndrome (MODS). This is evidenced by failure of the kidneys, cardiovascular system, and the presence of acute respiratory distress syndrome with sepsis. He is unresponsive to verbal and tactile stimuli on a ventilator with the following settings:

FIO_2	.80
Vt	600 ml
PEEP	10 cm H_2O
A/C	12 BPM

Which of the following interventions should the NP consider at this time?
   a. Call a conference with the health care team and family to discuss the decision for a DNR order for this patient.
   b. Order a stat consult with an infectious disease specialist to discuss additional antibiotics.
   c. Order a CT of the abdomen to determine if the bowel is healing.
   d. Give additional packed red blood cells to improve his volume.

SCENARIO 3

Questions 9–11 refer to the following scenario.

A patient reports to the ED with a chief complaint of chest tightness and air hunger. You note audible wheezes. Vital signs are HR = 108, RR = 28, Temp =

98.6°F, and B/P = 140/88. On examination, you find erythematous nasal passages, tender cervical adenopathy, coarse upper airway sounds with scattered rhonchi, and expiratory wheezes.

9. Which of the following is the most important piece of data that should be ordered at this time?
   a. An EKG and scheduling a stress test.
   b. A pulse oximeter reading and PFTs.
   c. A CBC and chemistry panel.
   d. A treatment with albuterol followed by acetylcysteine.

10. The remainder of this patient's exam is unremarkable. The SpO_2 is 95 percent on room air. The peak flow is 350. PFT data are as follows:

	Meas	Pred	% Pred
FVC	2.63	3.11	84
FEV1	1.58	2.28	69
FEV1/FVC	60	73	
FEC 25–75	0.59	2.56	32
PEF	4.90	5.78	85

This patient has been diagnosed with an acute bronchitis exacerbation. To improve the patient's respiratory efforts, you would:
   a. Order stat allergy testing.
   b. Draw ABGs.
   c. Start an aminophylline infusion.
   d. Administer nebulizer treatments × 3 using albuterol.

11. The albuterol resolves the wheezing but the patient continues to have some rhonchi on assessment. The chest X-ray reveals bronchitis in addition to the asthma. The SpO_2 remains 95 percent. Your discharge treatment plan should include:
   a. Contacting the family for additional information.
   b. Ordering a macrolide antibiotic and a short course of steroids with an albuterol MDI.
   c. Prescribing a Medrol dose pack and penicillin.
   d. Prescribing oxygen therapy for home use and contacting the family.

12. The nurse practitioner is managing a patient with acute respiratory distress syndrome. The patient is intubated and is on mechanical ventilation with the following settings:

FIO_2 1.0
Vt   600 ml
PEEP   10 cm H_2O
A/C   12 BPM

Vital signs are as follows:

B/P	90/50
HR	128
RR	32
Temp	98.6°F

A pulmonary artery catheter is in place. Data are:

PAP	42/24 mm Hg
PAWP	25 mm Hg
CVP	10 mm Hg

The intervention with the highest priority at this time is to:
    a. Order furosemide (Lasix®) 40 mg ×1.
    b. Insert a chest tube for the high PEEP levels.
    c. Notify the patient's family to determine the patient's advanced directives.
    d. Aggressively hydrate with crystalloids to combat third spacing in the lungs.

13. A patient with ARDS is on a mechanical ventilator. The patient has been provided adequate pulmonary toileting and pulmonary embolism has been ruled out. The patient is receiving PEEP of 12 cm and an FIO_2 of 1.0, but the SpO_2 drops from 92 percent to 70 percent. The patient's peak airway pressure increases from 36 to 80 cm H_2O. The immediate intervention of the nurse practitioner is to:
    a. Contact the pulmonologist.
    b. Order stat ABGs.
    c. Contact the family.
    d. Insert a chest tube.

SCENARIO 4

Questions 14–16 refer to the following scenario.

A 38-year-old African-American patient comes to see you, the NP, for a pre-employment physical examination. His history includes the following information: He is married with two children, ages 9 and 12; works as an account manager at a bank; has smoked one pack of cigarettes per day for the past 25 years; drinks 18 to 20 beers per week; and his diet is high in fat and carbohydrates. His family history includes diabetes, hypertension, and hypercholesterolemia. He describes himself as basically healthy with no specific health-related problems at this time except a great deal of stress on the job and at home trying to raise his children. Physical examination reveals: Ht: 6', Wt: 252 lbs, BP: 138/88; otherwise unremarkable.

14. According to Joint National Commission on Prevention, Detection, Evaluation and Blood Pressure Control (JNC 7) guidelines this man's BP is classified as:
    a. Stage I hypertension.
    b. Within normal limits.
    c. Mild hypertension.
    d. Prehypertension.

15. The best plan for the patient at this point would be:
    a. No treatment indicated at this time.
    b. Begin a thiazide diuretic.
    c. Initiate lifestyle modifications.
    d. Begin a beta blocker.

16. Patients who are at higher risk for sodium sensitivity include all of the following *except*:
    a. Older persons.
    b. African-Americans.
    c. Diabetics.
    d. Heart failure patients.

17. The goal for the patient's blood pressure is:
    a. <140/90.
    b. <130/80.
    c. <120/80.
    d. <130/85.

18. The patient returns for a third follow-up visit and his blood pressure is 142/100. Prior to initiating pharmacologic therapy, the NP would order which of the recommended laboratory tests according to JNC 7 guidelines?
    a. Blood chemistry, EKG, stress test, hemoglobin.
    b. BUN, U/A, echocardiogram, hemoglobin.
    c. Creatinine, U/A, echocardiogram, hemoglobin.
    d. Blood chemistry, 12–lead EKG, U/A, hematocrit.

19. The NP determines that it is necessary to begin pharmacologic therapy for the patient. In considering JNC 7 guidelines for initiation of an antihypertensive for this patient, the most appropriate choice would be:
    a. A diuretic and beta blocker.
    b. A diuretic and angiotensin receptor blocker.
    c. A diuretic and ACE inhibitor.
    d. A beta blocker and calcium channel blocker.

20. Compelling indications for the use of diuretics as antihypertensive treatment include all the following except:
    a. Heart failure.
    b. Post MI.
    c. Recurrent stroke prevention.
    d. Diabetes.

SCENARIO 5

Questions 21–25 refer to the following scenario.
A patient comes to you, the NP, for a follow-up of a fasting lipid panel drawn at her previous visit. She has smoked one pack of cigarettes per day for 30 years and does not drink alcohol. Her weight is 180 lbs, height 5'4", and BP is 130/80.

Her values are: Total cholesterol 230 mg/dL; LDL 150 mg/dL; HDL 35 mg/dL; and triglycerides 180 mg/dL.

21. Based on the recommendations of the National Cholesterol Education Program (NCEP) Adult Treatment Panel (ATP) III, the target for her LDL cholesterol is:
    a. <160.
    b. <140.
    c. <130.
    d. <120.

22. The ATP III recommends therapeutic lifestyle changes (TLC) for similar patients. Which of the following TLC is the first priority:
    a. Reduce intake of saturated fats and cholesterol.
    b. Smoking cessation.
    c. Increase regular physical activity.
    d. Reduce weight.

23. Which of the following lipid levels have been shown to correlate more strongly with CHD risk in women than in men?
    a. HDL and LDL.
    b. LDL and triglycerides.
    c. HDL and total cholesterol.
    d. HDL and triglycerides.

The patient returns for a 3-month follow-up visit. After therapeutic lifestyle changes (TLC) and smoking cessation, her lipid levels are somewhat lower but LDL and HDL are not within target range. Triglycerides remain unchanged.

24. According to NCEP ATPIII guidelines, the NP should:
    a. Continue TLC.
    b. Initiate statin therapy.
    c. Initiate a trial of niacin.
    d. Initiate fibrate therapy.

25. The patient's HDL level remains low at the next visit in another 3 months. The NP decides to add a niacin or fibrate. The choice of agent depends on:
    a. Triglyceride level.
    b. HDL level.
    c. LDL level.
    d. Total cholesterol.

ANSWER KEY AND RATIONALES TO ADVANCED PRACTICE SAMPLE QUESTIONS: ADULT NURSE PRACTITIONER

1. Answer c

At this time, the patient is highly vulnerable, complex, and unstable by virtue of being immediate postoperative state with several medical comorbidities in the reported history. The patient is also exhibiting a low level of resiliency by not developing compensatory mechanisms for the described condition. Ordering tests to check for platelets is the most important function at this time. This will address the high vulnerability and complexity of a problem that could be developing. With this intervention, the NP is demonstrating competency in clinical judgment by basing care on the immediate grasp of the whole picture of the patient. Choices a, b, and d do not describe interventions that are of higher priority. A determination needs to be made as to why the patient is bleeding prior to administering blood. Giving blood is not the immediate treatment. Although it is important to notify the family of a change in a patient's condition, this intervention does not address the patient's highly vulnerable state. Returning the patient to the operating room at this time is not the first line of treatment due to the patient's high vulnerability and low stability and the need to identify the underlying cause of the bleeding. Medical interventions may be required to remedy this situation.

REFERENCES

AACN. (2004). The AACN Synergy Model for Patient Care. Available at: http://www.aacn.org/certcorp.nsf/vwdoc/SynModel?opendocument. Accessed May 12, 2004.

Curley, M. A. Q. (1998). Patient-Nurse Synergy: Optimizing Patients' Outcomes. *American Journal of Critical Care* 7(1): 64–72.

Kaplow, R. (2003). AACN Synergy Model for Patient Care: A Framework to Optimize Outcomes. *Critical Care Nurse* 23(Suppl. 1): 27–30.

Kinney, M., Dunbar, S. B., Brooks-Brunn, J. A., Molter, N., and Vitello-Cicciu, J. M. (1998). *AACN: Clinical Reference for Critical Care Nursing*, 4th ed. (pp. 394–395). St. Louis, MO: C. V. Mosby Co.

2. Answer a

At this time, the patient continues to be highly vulnerable, complex, and unstable given the ongoing bleeding. The lab data do not suggest the source of the bleeding can be controlled with medical interventions. The patient is also exhibiting a low level of resiliency by not developing compensatory mechanisms for the described condition. The only way to stabilize the patient appears to be with a return to surgery. Notifying the family in choice b does not address the vulnerable state factor of this client as the immediate priority. Administering fresh frozen plasma in choice c will not resolve the instability or vulnerability issue of this patient as medical interventions do not appear indicated to eradicate the patient's clinical problem. Obtaining the lab data suggested in choice d will give some needed information but will not resolve the bleeding issue to address the high vulnerability and instability problem and will delay treatment of the likely underlying cause of the problem.

REFERENCES

AACN. (2004). The AACN Synergy Model for Patient Care. Available at: http://www.aacn.org/certcorp.nsf/vwdoc/SynModel?opendocument. Accessed May 12, 2004.

Curley, M. A. Q. (1998). Patient-Nurse Synergy: Optimizing Patients' Outcomes. *American Journal of Critical Care* 7(1): 64–72.

Kaplow, R. (2003). AACN Synergy Model for Patient Care: A Framework to Optimize Outcomes. *Critical Care Nurse* 23(Suppl. 1): 27–30.

Kinney, M., Dunbar, S. B., Brooks-Brunn, J. A., Molter, N., and Vitello-Cicciu, J. M. (1998). *AACN: Clinical Reference for Critical Care Nursing* 4th ed. (pp. 394–395). St. Louis, MO: C. V. Mosby Co.

3. Answer c

At this time, the patient continues to demonstrate low levels of resiliency and moderate levels of stability based on the elevated blood sugar. The high blood glucose needs to be addressed for the stability of the body with the effects of the glucose. Limiting activity, as suggested in choice a, will not address the issue of resiliency. Increasing activity as tolerated will assist with resiliency and participation in care. In choice b, a pulse rate of 60 does not address the body's ability to be resilient. In addition, a heart rate of 60 is often a resting heart rate, not one associated with activity.

Increasing the dose of oral agents, as indicated in choice d, does not address the complexity of the body to adjust to times of stress. In this situation, the NP is exhibiting competency in clinical judgment by making judgments based on an immediate grasp of the whole picture for a patient of a routine population. The NP is also exhibiting competency in collaboration by involving other resources; in this case the internal medicine provider, to optimize patient outcomes. The NP is not demonstrating competency as a facilitator of learning by not demonstrating a focus on the patient and not providing education to help resolve the problem.

REFERENCES

AACN. (2004). The AACN Synergy Model for Patient Care. Available at: http://www.aacn.org/certcorp.nsf/vwdoc/SynModel?opendocument. Accessed May 12, 2004.

Curley, M. A. Q. (1998). Patient-Nurse Synergy: Optimizing Patients' Outcomes. *American Journal of Critical Care* 7(1): 64–72.

Kaplow, R. (2003). AACN Synergy Model for Patient Care: A Framework to Optimize Outcomes. *Critical Care Nurse* 23(Suppl. 1): 27–30.

Kinney, M., Dunbar, S. B., Brooks-Brunn, J. A., Molter, N., and Vitello-Cicciu, J. M. (1998). *AACN: Clinical Reference for Critical Care Nursing* 4th ed. (pp. 391–395). St. Louis, MO: C. V. Mosby Co.

4. Answer a

At this time, the patient has moderate levels of vulnerability, being somewhat susceptible, and low levels of stability and resiliency by being unable to mount a compensatory response. By selecting the correct regimen, the NP is exhibiting competency in clinical judgment. The NP is making judgments based on an immediate grasp of the whole picture and is using past experiences and experiential knowledge to treat and anticipate problems. This regimen in choice a will address the stability, vulnerability, and resiliency of the patient. Regimens in the other three choices will not provide adequate stability and do not address all of the factors related to heart failure. This regimen is not recommended and will not provide for adequate resiliency because it does not address the preload/afterload issues associated with nitroglycerin.

REFERENCES

AACN. (2004). The AACN Synergy Model for Patient Care. Available at: http://www.aacn.org/certcorp.nsf/vwdoc/SynModel?opendocument. Accessed May 12, 2004.

Curley, M. A. Q. (1998). Patient-Nurse Synergy: Optimizing Patients' Outcomes. *American Journal of Critical Care* 7(1): 64–72.

Irwin, R., Cerra, F., and Rippe, J. (1999) *Intensive Care Medicine*, 4th ed. (pp. 465–468). Philadelphia: Lippincott, Williams & Wilkins.

Kaplow, R. (2003). AACN Synergy Model for Patient Care: A Framework to Optimize Outcomes. *Critical Care Nurse* 23(Suppl. 1): 27–30.

5. Answer a

In this situation, the patient is exhibiting moderate levels of vulnerability and stability, being somewhat susceptible, and has some degree of a steady state at this time. The NP is demonstrating competency in clinical judgment by basing care on the immediate grasp of the whole picture of the patient who is part of a common population. Due to the complexity of this patient and the metabolic acidosis that can occur as result of poor tissue perfusion, these tests address the issues of complexity, stability, and vulnerability of this patient. Laboratory tests in choice b do not take into practice all of the complications that could occur due to the complexity and vulnerability of this patient. The laboratory tests in choices c and d do not include the arterial blood gases. The lab findings received will not provide enough data to address the issues of stability and vulnerably.

REFERENCES

AACN. (2004). The AACN Synergy Model for Patient Care. Available at: http://www.aacn.org/certcorp.nsf/vwdoc/SynModel?opendocument. Accessed May 12, 2004.

Curley, M. A. Q. (1998). Patient-Nurse Synergy: Optimizing Patients' Outcomes. *American Journal of Critical Care* 7(1): 64–72.

Kaplow, R. (2003). AACN Synergy Model for Patient Care: A Framework to Optimize Outcomes. *Critical Care Nurse* 23(Suppl. 1): 27–30.

6. Answer a

Narrowing or blockage of one or more of the mesenteric arteries causes mesenteric ischemia. It can also be caused by a blood clot that travels through the bloodstream and blocks one of the mesenteric arteries. If a blood clot breaks away and travels through the bloodstream, acute mesenteric ischemia is life threatening because the blood flow to the intestine is cut off completely, which can cause the intestine to die if not treated immediately. At this time, the patient continues to exhibit moderate levels of stability but is highly vulnerable. Symptoms of acute mesenteric ischemia are usually nonspecific initially, and diagnosis and treatment are often delayed as a result. This patient is demonstrating signs of bowel becoming gangrenous with the rectal bleeding that has been taking place since admission to the ED. The patient must be stabilized with intravenous fluids. The NP is demonstrating competency in clinical judgment by basing care on the immediate grasp of the whole picture of the patient of a population that is not very common. The vulnerability and instability of this patient are the most serious issues to be addressed. An enterostomal therapist is not needed at this immediate time. The interventions in choices b, c, and d do not address the patient's emergent needs.

REFERENCES

AACN. (2004). The AACN Synergy Model for Patient Care. Available at: http://www.aacn.org/certcorp.nsf/vwdoc/SynModel?opendocument. Accessed May 12, 2004.

Curley, M. A. Q. (1998). Patient-Nurse Synergy: Optimizing Patients' Outcomes. *American Journal of Critical Care* 7(1): 64–72.

Dang, C., Wade, J., and Mandal, A. (2003). Acute Mesenteric Ischemia. Available at: http:// www.emedicine.com/med/topic 2627.htm. Accessed July 11, 2003.

Irwin, R., Cerra, F., and Rippe, J. (1999). *Intensive Care Medicine*, 4th ed. (pp. 1884–1885). Philadelphia: Lippincott, Williams & Wilkins.

Kaplow, R. (2003). AACN Synergy Model for Patient Care: A Framework to Optimize Outcomes. *Critical Care Nurse* 23(Suppl. 1): 27–30.

7. Answer b

Patients with acute mesenteric ischemia may require resection of necrotic bowel if signs of peritonitis develop. Given the patient's febrile state and presence of peritonitis is possible. Emergency surgical intervention is crucial if there is any chance of saving this patient. It is important to have the family come to the hospital, but this does not address the issue of high complexity and low stability for this patient. It is important to be aware of the spiritual needs of the patient, but this does not address the crucial issues of high complexity and low stability. Contacting the blood bank for a type and cross match is not the duty of the NP and does not meet the patient's current immediate needs.

REFERENCES

AACN. (2004). The AACN Synergy Model for Patient Care. Available at: http://www.aacn.org/certcorp.nsf/vwdoc/SynModel?opendocument. Accessed May 12, 2004.

Curley, M. A. Q. (1998). Patient-Nurse Synergy: Optimizing Patients' Outcomes. *American Journal of Critical Care* 7(1): 64–72.

Dang, C., Wade, J., & Mandal, A. (2003). Acute Mesenteric Ischemia. Available at: http:// www.emedicine.com/med/topic 2627.htm. Accessed July 11, 2003.

Irwin, R., Cerra, F., & Rippe, J. (1999). *Intensive Care Medicine* 4th ed. (pp. 1882–1886). Philadelphia: Lippincott, Williams & Wilkins.

Kaplow, R. (2003). AACN Synergy Model for Patient Care: A Framework to Optimize Outcomes. *Critical Care Nurse* 23(Suppl. 1): 27–30.

8. Answer a

A meeting with all members of the health care team and family would best address the medical and ethical concerns in this situation. In this situation, the patient is exhibiting high levels of complexity, vulnerability, and instability given the life-threatening condition. The patient is also exhibiting low levels of ability to participate in care or in decision making. The NP is demonstrating competency in caring practices by recognizing that death may be an acceptable outcome for the patient, and competency in collaboration by facilitating the active involvement and complementary contributions of other team members in the plan of care of this patient. The NP is also demonstrating competency in advocacy/moral agency by considering the family's values and incorporating them into the plan of care.

In this case, the plan of care requires an interdisciplinary team meeting with the family regarding the patient's status. The meeting will give the family an opportunity to speak and represent themselves and allow them to express what they know about the patient's wishes regarding care. The NP is also working on behalf of the patient and family by coordinating the meeting. With the status of the patient and his high complexity, the family has the capacity to assist in the decision making and resources to make an informed decision on this patient's life. An infectious disease specialist has likely been consulted given the need for antibiotics early in the patient's presentation. Even with the high complexity and minimal stability, consultation with an infectious disease specialist is not necessary at this time. Given the low levels of resiliency, predictability, and stability and the high level of vulnerability, additional diagnostic tests are not indicated at this time. It is time to use the decision making of the family for the good of the patient. Additional blood is not indicated at this time.

REFERENCES

AACN. (2004). The AACN Synergy Model for Patient Care. Available at: http:// www.aacn.org/certcorp.nsf/vwdoc/SynModel?opendocument. Accessed May 12, 2004.

Curley, M. A. Q. (1998). Patient-Nurse Synergy: Optimizing Patients' Outcomes. *American Journal of Critical Care* 7(1): 64–72.

Irwin, R., Cerra, F., & Rippe, J. (1999). *Intensive Care Medicine* 4th ed. (pp. 1882–1886). Philadelphia: Lippincott, Williams & Wilkins.

Kaplow, R. (2003). AACN Synergy Model for Patient Care: A Framework to Optimize Outcomes. *Critical Care Nurse* 23(Suppl. 1): 27–30.

9. Answer b

In this situation, the patient is exhibiting high levels of vulnerability, as evidenced by the susceptible, fragile status with air hunger and other respiratory symptomatology. The patient has a moderate level of stability and resiliency; her vital signs show the ability to maintain a steady state at this time and compensate for her condition. Choices a, c, and d do not address the findings and the vulnerability of this patient. The NP is exhibiting competency in clinical judgment by selecting the appropriate diagnostics by making judgment based on an immediate grasp of the whole picture for the patient in a routine population.

REFERENCES

AACN. (2004). The AACN Synergy Model for Patient Care. Available at: http://www.aacn.org/certcorp.nsf/vwdoc/SynModel?opendocument. Acessed May 12, 2004.

Curley, M. A. Q. (1998). Patient-Nurse Synergy: Optimizing Patients' Outcomes. *American Journal of Critical Care* 7(1): 64–72.

Kaplow, R. (2003). AACN Synergy Model for Patient Care: A Framework to Optimize Outcomes. *Critical Care Nurse* 23(Suppl. 1): 27–30.

Kinney, M., Dunbar, S. B., Brooks-Brunn, J. A., Molter, N., and Vitello-Cicciu, J. M. (1998). *AACN: Clinical Reference for Critical Care Nursing* 4th ed. (pp. 578–580). St. Louis, MO: C. V. Mosby Co.

10. Answer d

In this situation, the patient is exhibiting moderate levels of resiliency and stability and low levels of vulnerability. The patient is maintaining a steady state despite the presenting signs and symptoms. There is a low risk for death at this time. The patient is demonstrating high levels of participation in care by being able to assist in pulmonary function testing. Interventions in choices a, b, and c do not address the issue or diagnosis based on the patient's high resiliency and high stability. The NP is exhibiting competency in clinical judgment by demonstrating an immediate grasp of the whole picture and interpretation of data for a common patient population.

REFERENCES

AACN. (2004). The AACN Synergy Model for Patient Care. Available at: http://www.aacn.org/certcorp.nsf/vwdoc/SynModel?opendocument. Accessed May 12, 2004.

Curley, M. A. Q. (1998). Patient-Nurse Synergy: Optimizing Patients' Outcomes. *American Journal of Critical Care* 7(1): 64–72.

Kaplow, R. (2003). AACN Synergy Model for Patient Care: A Framework to Optimize Outcomes. *Critical Care Nurse* 23(Suppl. 1): 27–30.

Kinney, M., Dunbar, S. B., Brooks-Brunn, J. A., Molter, N., and Vitello-Cicciu, J. M. (1998). *AACN: Clinical Reference for Critical Care Nursing* 4th ed. (pp. 578–580). St. Louis, MO: C. V. Mosby Co.

11. Answer b

At this time, the patient is exhibiting high levels of resiliency and stability as evidenced by the plan for discharge. The patient has exhibited high levels of ability to participate in care. Choices a, c, and d are not interventions consistent with the patient characteristics described. The NP is exhibiting competency in clinical judgment by demonstrating an immediate grasp of the whole picture for a common patient population.

REFERENCES

AACN. (2004). The AACN Synergy Model for Patient Care. Available at: http:// www.aacn.org/certcorp.nsf/vwdoc/SynModel?opendocument. Accessed May 12, 2004.

Curley, M. A. Q. (1998). Patient-Nurse Synergy: Optimizing Patients' Outcomes. *American Journal of Critical Care* 7(1): 64–72.

Kaplow, R. (2003). AACN Synergy Model for Patient Care: A Framework to Optimize Outcomes. *Critical Care Nurse* 23(Suppl. 1): 27–30.

Kinney, M., Dunbar, S. B., Brooks-Brunn, J. A., Molter, N., & Vitello-Cicciu, J. M. (1998). *AACN: Clinical Reference for Critical Care Nursing* 4th ed. (pp. 578–580). St. Louis, MO: C. V. Mosby Co.

12. Answer a

In this situation, the patient is exhibiting high levels of vulnerability and low levels of stability and resiliency. Diuresing the patient will decrease the PAWP. With the high vulnerability and minimal stability, this is the best course of treatment. A chest tube is not indicated at this time because there is no evidence of a pneumothorax and it is not a procedure done on a prophylactic basis. The patient's family should be notified but this is not the immediate priority given the patient's levels of vulnerability and instability. Increasing fluid volume will only heighten the vulnerability and instability of this patient.

REFERENCES

AACN. (2004). The AACN Synergy Model for Patient Care. Available at: http://www.aacn.org/certcorp.nsf/vwdoc/SynModel?opendocument. Accessed May 12, 2004.

Curley, M. A. Q. (1998). Patient-Nurse Synergy: Optimizing Patients' Outcomes. *American Journal of Critical Care* 7(1): 64–72.

Irwin, R., Cerra, F., & Rippe, J. (1999). *Intensive Care Medicine* 4th ed. (pp. 584–590). Philadelphia: Lippincott, Williams & Wilkins.

Kaplow, R. (2003). AACN Synergy Model for Patient Care: A Framework to Optimize Outcomes. *Critical Care Nurse* 23(Suppl. 1): 27–30.

13. Answer d

This patient is in a state of minimal resiliency, high vulnerability, and minimal stability. There is no time to contact a pulmonologist when the nurse suspects that the patient has developed a pneumothorax. Emergent intervention is essential. ABG results will not provide any additional information to help correct this problem. The family should be contacted but emergent treatment of the pneumothorax is the first priority.

REFERENCES

Curley, M. A. Q. (1998). Patient-Nurse Synergy: Optimizing Patients' Outcomes. *American Journal of Critical Care* 7(1): 64–72.

Irwin, R., Cerra, F., & Rippe, J. (1999). *Intensive Care Medicine* 4th ed. (pp. 584–590). Philadelphia: Lippincott, Williams & Wilkins.

Kaplow, R. (2003). AACN Synergy Model for Patient Care: A Framework to Optimize Outcomes. *Critical Care Nurse* 23(Suppl. 1): 27–30.

14. Answer d

This is a new classification of hypertensive staging released by the Joint National Commission on Prevention, Detection, Evaluation and Blood Pressure Control (JNC 7) in May 2003. The latest guidelines are a result of clinical trials and observational studies from January 1997 until April 2003. Research also demonstrated that providers are not using the new guidelines. The most dramatic change in the new guidelines is the addition of the prehypertensive stage. Persons in the prehypertensive stage were twice as likely to become hypertensive as those with lower values. The patient is in a vulnerable state and susceptible to stressors that may adversely affect his health if interventions are not taken at this point. The NP's response to diversity will allow her to recognize that African-Americans are more susceptible to this disease and allow her to make appropriate clinical judgments for this patient. The NP is using evidence-based standards to accurately categorize the patient. In this manner, the nurse practitioner is demonstrating competency in clinical inquiry.

REFERENCES

Chobanian, A.V., Bakris, G. L., Black, H. R., Cushman, W. C., Green, L. A., Izzo, J. L., Jr., Jones, D. W., Materson, B. J., Oparil, S., Wright, J. T., Jr., & Roccella, E. J.; National Heart, Lung, and Blood Institute Joint National Committee on

Prevention, Detection, Evaluation, and Treatment of High Blood Pressure; National High Blood Pressure Education Program Coordinating Committee. (2003). The Seventh Report of the Joint National Committee on Prevention, Detection, Evaluation, and Treatment of High Blood Pressure: The JNC 7 Report. *Journal of the American Medical Association* 289(19): 2560–2572.

Lookinland, S., & Beckstrand, R. (2003). Evidence-Based Treatment of Hypertension. *Advance for Nurse Practitioners* 11(9): 32–40.

15. Answer c

For the prehypertensive stage, lifestyle modifications of decreased dietary sodium, the Dietary Approach to Stopping Hypertension (DASH), decreased alcohol ingestion, smoking cessation, and exercise should be initiated. As a facilitator of learning for the patient and family, the NP will coordinate a comprehensive program of lifestyle modifications, collaborating with the necessary resources to accomplish the goals mutually agreed upon. The nurse practitioner is demonstrating competency in clinical judgment and clinical inquiry in this situation.

REFERENCES

Lookinland, S., & Beckstrand, R. (2003). Evidence-Based Treatment of Hypertension. *Advance for Nurse Practitioners* 11(9): 32–40.

Vidt, D. G., & Borazanian, R. A. (2003). Treat High Blood Pressure Sooner: Tougher, Simpler JNC 7 Guidelines. *The Cleveland Clinic Journal of Medicine* 70(8): 721–728.

16. Answer d

In research looking at the relationship between intake of dietary sodium and hypertension, certain groups have been determined as salt sensitive. These include older persons, African-Americans, and diabetics. The NP recognizes that these groups have threats to their stability and as a facilitator of learning, she will instruct these vulnerable groups on the principles of low sodium diets and monitor their capacity to initiate and maintain lifestyle changes. The NP is demonstrating competency in clinical judgment and clinical inquiry by basing care on the immediate grasp of the whole picture of the patient and implementing evidence-based standards of care.

REFERENCES

Lookinland, S., & Beckstrand, R. (2003). Evidence-Based Treatment of Hypertension. *Advance for Nurse Practitioners* 11(9): 32–40.

Grimm, R. (2001). Cardiovascular Risk Factor Management. *Therapeutic Spotlight: A Supplement to Clinician Reviews* (pp. 3–12). New York: Jobson Publishers.

17. Answer c

According to JNC 7 guidelines, a BP <120/80 significantly reduces cardiovascular events. The risk of CVD for those with BPs > 115/75 doubles for every increment of 20/10 mm Hg. The NP demonstrates competency in clinical inquiry by basing the assessment of the patient and decision making on research-based evidence from national standards of care.

REFERENCES

Lookinland, S., & Beckstrand, R. (2003). Evidence-Based Treatment of Hypertension. *Advance for Nurse Practitioners* 11(9): 32–40.
van Vlaanderen, E. (2003). New Hypertension Guidelines. *The Clinical Advisor* 12(6): 13–16.

18. Answer d

These laboratory tests are recommended to determine pretherapy values and detect causes of secondary hypertension. These tests also most accurately assess target organ damage. Hematocrit assesses anemia and polycythemia; blood glucose to assess for diabetes and pheochromocytoma; potassium for hyperaldosteronism, sodium to assess volume status, creatinine for renal insufficiency, a total lipid panel to assess vessel status; a urinalysis to assess for hematuria, proteinuria, and casts; and an EKG to guide medication selection. If a person has peaked T waves from hyperkalemia, the NP should not prescribe ACE inhibitors or potassium-sparing diuretics because these drugs can increase potassium levels that may result in life-threatening complications. Again the NP uses the dimension of clinical inquiry in using evidence-based research to order the most appropriate lab tests. Using the most cost effective measures without compromising quality patient care recognizes that the NP is part of a health care system and appreciates the constraints of the particular environment such as managed care. The NP is demonstrating systems thinking.

REFERENCES

Huffstutler, S. (2000). Managing Hypertension in African-American Men. *Advance for Nurse Practitioners* 8(4): 18–24.
Lookinland, S., & Beckstrand, R. (2003). Evidence-Based Treatment of Hypertension. *Advance for Nurse Practitioners* 11(9): 32–40.

19. Answer d

African-Americans have a higher prevalence of hypertension and are at high risk of hypertensive complications. Physiologic characteristics that contribute to that risk include low circulating renin with excessive levels of angiotensin II, more likely to be salt sensitive, and higher levels of intracellular calcium stores. Diuretics are considered the initial drug of choice of uncomplicated hypertension.

Because of the higher prevalence of hypertension among African-Americans, few can reach target blood pressure with a single drug. All antihypertensive drugs lower blood pressure in the population if adequately dosed. However, JNC 7 recommends that diuretics and calcium channel blockers be considered the initial drugs of choice. Clinical inquiry and clinical judgment are essential NP characteristics for providing the most up-to-date research-based care. This also illustrates the NP using caring practices to respond to the uniqueness of this African-American patient.

REFERENCES

Huffstutler, S. (2000). Managing Hypertension in African-American Men. *Advance for Nurse Practitioners* 8(4): 18–24.
Lookinland, S., & Beckstrand, R. (2003). Evidence-Based Treatment of Hypertension. *Advance for Nurse Practitioners* 11(9): 32–40.

20. Answer b

Low doses of diuretics are safe and useful for diabetics because they act synergistically with other drugs, minimize electrolyte abnormalities, and reduce fluid retention common in diabetics. Thiazide diuretics are the first line agents for treatment of hypertension in African-Americans. Beta blockers are the preferred drug of choice for patients with previous MI. The NP recognizes the importance of cultural uniqueness in the application of research-based plans of care. In this situation, the NP is demonstrating competency in response to diversity and clinical inquiry.

REFERENCES

Huffstutler, S. (2000). Managing Hypertension in African-American Men. *Advance for Nurse Practitioners* 8(4): 18–24.
Lookinland, S., and Beckstrand, R. (2003). Evidence-Based Treatment of Hypertension. *Advance for Nurse Practitioners* 11(9): 32–40.

21. Answer a

According to ATP III guidelines, recommended LDL cholesterol goals for a patient with 0-1 risk factor is less than 160. The only risk factor in this patient thus far is smoking. Current ATP III guidelines focus on a more intensive approach to primary prevention. The use of clinical inquiry enables the NP to search and use research-based evidence and evaluate its appropriateness for unique individuals. As an advocate for women's health care, the NP recognizes that women are vulnerable to heart disease and have their stability threatened.

REFERENCE

McBride, P. (2003). The Importance of Risk Assessment in Identifying Patients at High Cardiovascular Risk. *Consultant* 43(14): 54–57.

22. Answer b

The risk priority for this patient is smoking cessation which will lower CHD risk and improve her lipid profile. It is important to tell this patient to see a dietitian and engage in regular exercise because smoking cessation may cause her to gain weight. The NP recognizes that the patient's stability is threatened by this particular unhealthy behavior and CHD risk factor. Using clinical judgment based on the evidence, the NP decides to strongly encourage the patient to enroll in a smoking cessation program. Through her caring practices, she monitors the patient's progress and encourages her along the way by a carefully implemented program of systematic follow-up. As a facilitator of learning, the NP is also able to recommend effective strategies and community resources to accomplish this goal.

REFERENCE

Mosca, L. (2003). Primary Prevention of CHD in Women. *Consultant* 43(14): 513–516.

23. Answer b

Both HDL and triglyceride levels have been shown in multiple studies to correlate more strongly with CHD risk in women than men. According to one meta-analysis, a 1-mmol/L increase was associated with a 31 percent increase in CHD risk in men and a 76 percent increase in women. In another report conducted by the National Heart and Lung and Blood Institute, HDL was reported to significantly relate with CHD events in middle aged and elderly women and was a stronger predictor more so in women than men 65 years or older. As a member of a vulnerable group, it is important that this patient be carefully followed and monitored. The NP knows that there are differences in risk factors, patterns of CHD, and treatment for women and that recent research has focused more on women and heart disease. As advocates and moral agents, NPs must continue to advocate for well-designed studies of women and CHD.

REFERENCE

Austin, M. (1999). Epidemiology of Hypertriglyceridemia and Cardiovascular Disease. *American Journal of Cardiology* 88: 13–16.

24. Answer b

Statins are the first line of therapy. They are the most effective agents for lower LDL and have been shown to seriously reduce CHD risk in multiple randomized clinical trials. Studies have shown that statins reduce LDL by 28 percent, triglycerides by 13 percent, and increased HDL by 5 percent. The NP uses clinical inquiry and judgment to design the most appropriate plan of care for this patient.

REFERENCE

Mosca, L. (2003). Primary Prevention of CHD in Women. *Consultant* 43(14): 513–516.

25. Answer a

The triglyceride level may help decide between niacin and a fibrate. If triglycerides are lower than 200 mg/dL, then niacin is the better choice because it is the most effective agent for raising HDL and is also effective in lowering triglycerides. If triglycerides are greater than 200 mg/dL, add a fibrate because these agents are particularly effective in lowering triglyceride levels. Evaluating the options for effective treatment is essential to the role of the NP. Using the Synergy Model as a guide can help the NP provide a holistic plan of care for this patient including lifestyle changes and the most effective treatments for women who have special needs in relation to CHD, but who can return to stability when the NP designs a plan of care based on current guidelines and research.

REFERENCE

Mosca, L. (2003). Primary Prevention of CHD in Women. *Consultant* 43(14): 513–516.

CHAPTER 22

ADVANCED PRACTICE SAMPLE QUESTIONS: CLINICAL NURSE SPECIALIST

Roberta Kaplow, PhD, RN, CCNS, CCRN

INTRODUCTION

The following questions have been developed to provide examples of questions that integrate the patient and clinical nurse specialist (CNS) characteristics of the Synergy Model. The scenarios and questions in this chapter focus on the role of the CNS in a variety of patient care settings. Each question is followed by four choices. One answer is the best answer. An annotated key at the end of the questions provides the correct choice along with a rationale for why the other choices are not the best, based on the Synergy Model.

1. A nurse is caring for an Asian American for the first time. The nurse reports to you, the CNS, that the husband would not make eye contact while being updated on his wife's poor condition and prognosis. The CNS is concerned that the husband is not willing to listen or accept the information. The best intervention indicated for the CNS would be to:
   a. Consult with the social worker or case manager to increase family participation in care.
   b. Collaborate with the intensive care physician to have the critical care team speak with the husband.
   c. Check with the nurse manager to reassign the patient to a nurse of Asian descent.
   d. Explain that this is normal behavior for the culture when with strangers and provide cultural diversity information.

2. A patient with hypovolemic shock in the ICU is receiving aggressive fluid resuscitation with 0.9% normal saline. Which of the following acid-base disturbances would you, the CNS, instruct the nurse caring for the patient to observe for with this therapy?

    a. Metabolic acidosis.
    b. Metabolic alkalosis.
    c. Respiratory acidosis.
    d. Respiratory alkalosis.

3. Mr. C is a patient status post cardiac transplantation who is being discharged to the telemetry unit in the morning. Upon expressing concern about his readiness for transfer, you would:
    a. Assure him that he will be fine.
    b. Tell him that all patients feel the same way and that these feelings are normal.
    c. Collaborate with the cardiac surgeon to reaffirm Mr. C's readiness for discharge.
    d. Provide an accepting atmosphere to facilitate the patient's discussion of concerns.

4. Mr. C's family verbalizes concern about mood swings the patient has been experiencing since surgery. They state "he just isn't the same. This surgery was a mistake." Your best response would be to:
    a. Collaborate with the intensivist to request a psychiatric evaluation.
    b. Evaluate the patient for other signs of graft rejection.
    c. Explain that the mood swings are likely steroid induced.
    d. Discuss Mr. C's desire for more independence with him.

SCENARIO 1

Questions 5–7 refer to the following scenario.

    A patient with a history of Type I insulin-dependent diabetes is admitted to your unit with a diagnosis of diabetic ketoacidosis. As the CNS, you are overseeing the care being administered by a nurse newer to critical care. Lab values on admission are as follows:

pH 7.12	Na 126
pCO 20	K 6.1
pO_2 85	Cl 93
SaO_2 93%	CO_2 7
HCO_3 5	Glucose 570
Vital signs:	B/P 84/46
	HR 124
	RR 26
	Temp 98.6°

5. Which of the following is *not* indicated at this time?
    a. 50 units regular insulin IV push.
    b. 1 mEq/kg $NaHCO_3$ IV push.
    c. 15 mm NaPhos IVPB over 4 hours.
    d. NS at 200 ml/hour.

6. The patient received insulin to decrease the blood sugar and had labs monitored every 2 hours. Four hours later, lab values are as follows:

pH	7.22	Na 130	
pCO_2	21	K 4.9	
pO_2	95	Cl 96	
SaO_2	96%	CO_2 9	
HCO_3	10	Glucose 466	
Vital signs:	B/P 92/60		
	HR 100		
	RR 22		
	Temp 98.6°		

Which of the following is indicated at this time?
   a. Furosemide 20 mg IV push
   b. KPO_4 15 mm
   c. Dopamine infusion at 5 mcg/kg/min
   d. $NaHCO_3$ 1 mEq/kg

7. One hour later, labs are as follows:

Na	132
K	4.8
Cl	96
CO_2	10
Glucose	294

Which of the following is indicated at this time?
   a. NS at 100 ml/hour.
   b. Lantus® (insulin glargine) 0.3 IU/kg subcutaneously.
   c. D_5NS at 150 ml/hour.
   d. Glucophage® (metformin hcl) 500 mg po.

8. In anticipation of a new patient population being admitted to your unit, you are developing an in-service about postoperative management of patients status post liver transplantation. Management of which of the following would be included?
   a. Metabolic alkalosis.
   b. Hyponatremia.
   c. Hyperkalemia.
   c. Hypercalcemia.

9. As the CNS, you are precepting a new critical care nurse who is caring for a patient status post liver transplantation. Upon the patient being told that he is being transferred out of the ICU, the patient appears elated and euphoric. At this time, you would:
   a. Focus care primarily on the physiologic aspects because the patient does not feel the need to ventilate her feelings.
   b. Note that depression is unlikely to develop upon transfer.
   c. Collaborate with the intensivist to have a psych evaluation done as this is not a normal response.
   d. Assist the patient to set realistic goals.

10. You are developing an in-service session on disseminated intravascular coagulation (DIC). Which of the following is an associated pulmonary symptom you would include?
   a. Decreased pulmonary artery pressure
   b. Respiratory alkalosis
   c. Increased peak inspiratory pressure
   d. Bradypnea

11. A patient on your unit describes feelings of being held prisoner and dreaming about death. As the CNS, you would best assist the patient by:
   a. Assisting the primary nurse to schedule activities and encourage adherence to it.
   b. Limit visiting hours to put the patient on a routine.
   c. Provide the patient with attainable goals.
   d. Frequently orient the patient to his surroundings.

12. A patient with acute mitral stenosis is admitted to your unit with hemodynamic instability. Upon insertion of a pulmonary artery catheter, which of the following would you anticipate?
   a. Decreased LVEDP
   b. Decreased pulmonary artery pressures
   c. Decreased left atrial pressure
   d. Decreased c wave

13. An orientee asks you about heart sounds to expect in a patient with mitral stenosis. Your best response is:
   a. S3 gallop
   b. Rumbling apical systolic murmur
   c. S4 gallop
   d. Loud atrial first sound

14. A patient recently admitted to your unit has a diagnosis of acute respiratory insufficiency. The patient verbalizes feelings of strangeness and unreality and that she feels "less than a person." The nurse caring for the patient asks you, as the CNS, how to manage this situation. The best response is:
   a. Engage the patient in the medically oriented conversation.
   b. Refer to the patient by her preferred name.
   c. Inform the patient of tests and procedures immediately before they are performed.
   d. Explain aspects of the environment to the patient, including the staff's names and responsibilities.

15. You are caring for a patient with multiple organ dysfunction syndrome who has undergone a liver resection to remove a tumor. The patient has a tracheostomy for prolonged need for mechanical ventilation, a feeding tube, and remains jaundiced. His face and extremities are edematous due

to aggressive fluid resuscitation required to support his blood pressure. The patient's wife requests permission to allow their 6-year-old son to visit. Your best response is to:

a. Explain that visiting in the ICU will expose the child to experiences he will not be able to cope with.

b. Explain that child visitation is against hospital policy and reassure her that the situation the patient is in is worse than the son could imagine it being.

c. Speak with the son in language understandable as to why he isn't allowed to visit his father.

d. Ask the patient and child if they want the visit to take place; if both agree, allow the visit to occur.

16. A patient, status post cardiopulmonary arrest due to acute myocardial infarction, is admitted to the ICU after successful resuscitation. The patient's wife verbalizes apprehension about him being left alone and is worried about a recurrent cardiac arrest. The best intervention would be to:

a. Encourage the wife to mourn with respect to her husband's dysfunction.

b. Enroll the patient in cardiac rehabilitation and survivor support group when he is discharged.

c. Provide literature to the family about cardiopulmonary resuscitation techniques.

d. Allow the wife to further express her feelings about the event.

17. A patient in your unit develops supraventricular tachycardia (SVT) with a rate of 236 that is refractory to pharmacological intervention. The physician suggests overdrive pacing. Because this is rarely done in the unit, the nurse caring for the patient seeks your assistance. What rate should be initially attempted?

a. 60

b. 100

c. 50

d. Patient's baseline heart rate on admission

18. A new nurse is caring for a patient with a history of coronary artery disease and ischemic cardiomyopathy. The patient is experiencing chest pain refractory to intravenous nitroglycerin. Intraaortic balloon counterpulsation is being considered. Which of the following would you suggest the nurse check for in the patient's history before assisting with this procedure?

a. Left bundle branch block

b. Aortic aneurysm

c. Congestive heart failure

d. Atherosclerosis

19. A nurse is floated from the postanesthesia care unit (PACU) to the ICU and is assigned a patient status post femoral popliteal bypass for whom perfusion has been successfully restored. Administration of which of the following should be anticipated?
   a. Sodium bicarbonate
   b. Potassium supplementation
   c. Acetazolamide (Diamox®)
   d. FFP with coagulation factors

20. A nurse expresses concern over continuing futile therapies for a patient under her care. You would:
   a. Question the family as to why they want to continue therapy.
   b. Check for a DNR order in the chart.
   c. Assist the RN to clarify the position of the stakeholders.
   d. Call the intensivist to address the issue.

21. A new graduate working in your ICU is caring for a patient who has a DNR order. The patient is on the ventilator with the following settings:

   FIO_2 .50
   Assist/Control Rate 12
   PEEP 5 cm
   Flow-by: ON

ABG results are as follows:

   pH 7.32
   pCO_2 50
   pO_2 58
   SaO_2 88%
   HCO_3 22

The physician orders read to decrease the A/C rate by 2 bpm and FIO_2 by 5 percent. You would instruct the nurse caring for the patient to:
   a. Speak with the family about the ventilator changes to keep them up-to-date.
   b. Call the respiratory therapist to make the ventilator changes.
   c. Collaborate with the physician regarding the rationale for the changes.
   d. Carry out the order to avoid disciplinary action.

22. A nurse new to critical care is taking care of a patient on strict isolation precautions. The physician enters the room without taking appropriate precautions. The nurse consults with you, the CNS, about what to do. You would instruct the nurse to:
   a. Report the physician to the intensivist.
   b. Instruct the physician to change clothing before entering other patients' rooms.
   c. Ask the physician to step outside the room and don appropriate garb.
   d. Place a yellow isolation tag on the physician upon exit from the patient's room.

23. You are caring for a patient whose clinical condition has dramatically deteriorated. The family members are divided about signing of a DNR order and are fighting in the waiting room. These disturbances are upsetting to other families in the waiting area and several other visitors come to you to complain. You would:
    a. Forbid the upset family from remaining in the waiting room.
    b. Arrange a family meeting for them to express their feelings.
    c. Set limits with the family regarding their behavior.
    d. Collaborate with the social worker to speak with the family.

24. A nurse is caring for a patient with unilateral lung disease. The nurse is working unassisted to position the patient with the diseased lung up. You would initially:
    a. Assist the nurse and encourage future use of help and good body mechanics.
    b. Encourage the nurse to position the patient on the opposite side.
    c. Leave research-based articles on management of unilateral lung disease for the nurse.
    d. Assist the nurse to perform chest physiotherapy and postural drainage.

25. A patient is admitted to the ICU status post motor vehicle crash. The patient sustained multiple internal injuries and is hemodynamically unstable upon admission to the ICU. The family arrives and is visibly concerned about the patient. You overhear the nurse caring for the patient tell the family that the patient is critically ill and that visiting hours start at midday the next day. You would initially:
    a. Ask the RN to explain why the family was sent home.
    b. Encourage the family to insist on visiting with the patient.
    c. Collaborate with the intensivist to change the visiting policy.
    d. Encourage the nurse to allow the family to visit for a short period, citing value from research studies.

ANSWER KEY AND RATIONALES TO ADVANCED PRACTICE SAMPLE QUESTIONS: CLINICAL NURSE SPECIALIST

1. Answer d

In this situation, the patient is exhibiting low levels of resiliency and high levels of vulnerability as evidenced by her poor condition. She has low levels of stability, as she does not appear to be responding to therapies, and low levels of predictability. She has moderate to high levels of resource availability, as evidenced by her husband visiting. The patient's spouse has moderate to high levels of vulnerability because his wife is seriously ill with a poor prognosis.

In this situation, the CNS is demonstrating competencies as an advocate and moral agent by trying to resolve clinical concerns of the patient and family. The

CNS is also acting as a facilitator of learning by providing an update on the patient's clinical status while being sensitive to the cultural diversity issues of the patient and family. The CNS is also demonstrating caring practices by helping to create a caring, compassionate, and therapeutic environment for the husband to be updated on his wife's status. Finally, the CNS is exhibiting response to diversity by recognizing and appreciating cultural differences into the provision of care.

Choices a, b, and c do not address the cultural preferences of the patient and family or speak to the issue of concern in the scenario. Choice c, reassigning a nurse of Asian descent to the patient, could possibly help in the situation if the new nurse was knowledgeable of the cultural differences being observed in the scenario.

REFERENCES

Curley, M. A. Q. (1998). Patient-Nurse Synergy: Optimizing Patients' Outcomes. *American Journal of Critical Care* 7(1): 64–72.

Kaplow, R. (2003). AACN Synergy Model for Patient Care: A Framework to Optimize Outcomes. *Critical Care Nurse* 23(Suppl. 1): 27–30.

Kirkwood, N. A. (1996). *A Hospital Handbook on Multiculturalism and Religion.* Alexandria, New South Wales, Australia: Millennium Books.

2. Answer a

In this situation, the patient has a low level of stability (requiring aggressive fluid resuscitation to sustain adequate perfusion), a high level of vulnerability (being susceptible to consequences of therapies or hypoperfusion), and a moderate level of predictability. These are evidenced by the clinical situation described.

In massive amounts, normal saline can cause hypokalemia, hypernatremia, and hyperchloremic acidosis. The latter serves to worsen the acidotic state that can develop in hypovolemic shock. This occurs because the high concentration of chloride ions in normal saline causes bicarbonate ions to be released in the kidney tubules, thus lowering the bicarbonate level in the extracellular fluid.

In this situation, the CNS is demonstrating high levels of clinical judgment as a global grasp of the situation is apparent. Choices b, c, and d are incorrect from a physiologic perspective.

REFERENCES

Curley, M. A. Q. (1998). Patient-Nurse Synergy: Optimizing Patients' Outcomes. *American Journal of Critical Care* 7(1): 64–72.

Kaplow, R. (2003). AACN Synergy Model for Patient Care: A Framework to Optimize Outcomes. *Critical Care Nurse* 23(Suppl. 1): 27–30.

Roberts, M. K. (1990). Hypovolemic Shock. In B. C. Mims, ed. *Case Studies in Critical Care Nursing* (p. 87). Baltimore, MD: Williams & Wilkins.

3. Answer d

In this situation, the patient is demonstrating high levels of predictability, stability, and resiliency. This is evidenced by the clearance for discharge from the intensive care unit. The patient's level of vulnerability is moderate from a psychological perspective and the level of participating in decision making is low in relation to transfer from the intensive care unit. The CNS, with the appropriate intervention, is acting as an advocate and moral agent by working on the patient's behalf and representing the patient's concerns. The CNS is also demonstrating caring practices. This is evidenced by the attempt to create a therapeutic environment and trying to promote emotional comfort in response to the patient's concerns regarding transfer from the intensive care unit.

The ICU patient experiences transfer anxiety when being moved from a familiar, relatively secure environment to a less familiar situation. It can result from the patient's lack of control over the determination of when they will be transferred out of the ICU. With the suddenness of the transfer, patients may not have the necessary time to understand the positive reasons for this change in environment.

Choice a is providing the patient with false reassurance, because there is no way to predict that the patient will not suffer any consequences following transfer. While acknowledging the patient's feelings and providing reassurance that the feelings are "normal" in Choice b, this is not completely addressing the patient's concerns. Choice c is not completely addressing the patient's concerns either because patients are traditionally transferred from the ICU following transplant based on a clinical pathway. It is likely that transfer orders were not written unless the patient was stable and ready from a physiologic perspective.

REFERENCES

Curley, M. A. Q. (1998). Patient-Nurse Synergy: Optimizing Patients' Outcomes. *American Journal of Critical Care* 7(1): 64–72.

Kaplow, R. (2003). AACN Synergy Model for Patient Care: A Framework to Optimize Outcomes. *Critical Care Nurse* 23(Suppl. 1): 27–30.

McHugh, L. G., Clark, K. G., and Pierson, D. J. (1992). Psychosocial Aspects of Critical Care: The Patient, the Family, the Staff. Patient Interactions. In D. J. Pierson and R. M. Kacmarek, eds. *Foundations of Respiratory Care* (pp. 1221–1236). New York: Churchill Livingstone.

4. Answer c

In this situation, the patient is stabilizing, has a moderate degree of vulnerability, a high degree of predictability, and a high degree of resource availability, as evidenced by the apparent concern about the patient's condition by the wife. The CNS, choosing the appropriate intervention, is demonstrating high levels of clinical judgment and caring practices and is acting as a facilitator of learning.

Mood swings are an anticipated side effect of steroid therapy. Acknowledging the symptoms and providing support to the patient and family is indicated at this time. A psychiatric evaluation is not necessarily indicated. Discussing Mr. C's desire for increasing independence will not address the family's concerns.

Choice a is not correct because a psychiatric evaluation is not clearly indicated in this instance. Mr. C is not exhibiting signs of graft rejection, as suggested in Choice b. Choice d does not address the issue described.

REFERENCES

Curley, M. A. Q. (1998). Patient-Nurse Synergy: Optimizing Patients' Outcomes. *American Journal of Critical Care* 7(1): 64–72.

Kaplow, R. (2003). AACN Synergy Model for Patient Care: A Framework to Optimize Outcomes. *Critical Care Nurse* 23(Suppl. 1): 27–30.

5. Answer b

In this situation, by selecting the correct answer, the CNS is exhibiting clinical judgment and caring practices. The patient is exhibiting high levels of vulnerability and complexity and low levels of stability given the critical nature of his illness at this time.

There is a decreased level of 2,3-DPG with diabetic ketoacidosis. This results in a shift to the left of the oxyhemoglobin dissociation curve, resulting in impaired dissociation of oxygen molecules from hemoglobin at the tissue level. In diabetic ketoacidosis, there is a shift to the right of the oxyhemoglobin dissociation curve due to a decrease in pH. The shifts counteract each other. Sodium bicarbonate administration should be reserved for circumstances when the patient's pH is < 6.9 to 7.0.

REFERENCES

Curley, M. A. Q. (1998). Patient-Nurse Synergy: Optimizing Patients' Outcomes. *American Journal of Critical Care* 7(1): 64–72.

Kaplow, R. (2003). AACN Synergy Model for Patient Care: A Framework to Optimize Outcomes. *Critical Care Nurse* 23(Suppl. 1): 27–30.

Roberts, M. K. (1990). Hypovolemic Shock. In B. C. Mims, ed. *Case Studies in Critical Care Nursing* (p. 357). Baltimore, MD: Williams & Wilkins.

6. Answer b

In this situation, the patient continues to exhibit high levels of vulnerability and complexity and low levels of stability. The patient is exhibiting moderate levels of predictability as the clinical responses to therapies administered were expected. By selecting the correct answer, the CNS continues to exhibit high levels of clinical judgment and caring practices.

Phosphorus is lost in urine due to osmotic diuresis from the hyperglycemia. In addition, phosphorus is required for glucose metabolism. Therefore, as insulin is given and metabolism is restored, serum phosphorus levels decrease even further. Phosphorus is required for the production of 2,3-DPG. If the patient develops hypophosphatemia, a shift to the left of the oxyhemoglobin dissociation curve will result. This can cause cellular oxygen deprivation.

REFERENCES

Curley, M. A. Q. (1998). Patient-Nurse Synergy: Optimizing Patients' Outcomes. *American Journal of Critical Care* 7(1): 64–72.

Jones, T. L. (1990). *Diabetic Ketoacidosis.* In B. C. Mims, ed. *Case Studies in Critical Care Nursing* (p. 359). Baltimore, MD: Williams & Wilkins.

Kaplow, R. (2003). AACN Synergy Model for Patient Care: A Framework to Optimize Outcomes. *Critical Care Nurse* 23(Suppl. 1): 27–30.

7. Answer c

In this situation, the patient is now stabilizing, is less vulnerable, and has demonstrated a high degree of predictability. The CNS, by selecting the correct option, is demonstrating a high level of clinical judgment and caring practices.

The patient's blood glucose level is normalizing; hence, there is a risk of precipitating hypoglycemia and subsequent cerebral edema. Choice a is incorrect because when a patient's blood sugar reaches 300 mg/dl, dextrose should be added to the intravenous fluids. Additional regular insulin should be given until the patient's anion gap, currently at 26 (132 − [96 + 10]) is minimized. Choices b and d are incorrect because neither therapy will lower blood sugar levels correctly based on their respective onsets of action.

REFERENCES

Curley, M. A. Q. (1998). Patient-Nurse Synergy: Optimizing Patients' Outcomes. *American Journal of Critical Care* 7(1): 64–72.

Jones, T. L. (1990). D*iabetic Ketoacidosis.* In B. C. Mims, ed. *Case Studies in Critical Care Nursing* (p. 360). Baltimore, MD: Williams & Wilkins.

Kaplow, R. (2003). AACN Synergy Model for Patient Care: A Framework to Optimize Outcomes. *Critical Care Nurse* 23(Suppl. 1): 27–30.

8. Answer a

In this situation, the CNS is demonstrating clinical judgment and acting as a facilitator of learning.

A metabolic alkaosis results from increased sodium retention and bicarbonate reabsorption by the kidneys. Hypokalemia results from renal loss of potassium and donor potassium uptake. The metabolic alkalosis is also due to metabolism of the blood preservative sodium citrate into bicarbonate as the new liver starts to function.

REFERENCES

Curley, M. A. Q. (1998). Patient-Nurse Synergy: Optimizing Patients' Outcomes. *American Journal of Critical Care* 7(1): 64–72.

Glass, C. (1990). *Liver Transplantation.* In B. C. Mims, ed. *Case Studies in Critical Care Nursing* (p. 391). Baltimore, MD: Williams & Wilkins.

Kaplow, R. (2003). AACN Synergy Model for Patient Care: A Framework to Optimize Outcomes. *Critical Care Nurse* 23(Suppl. 1): 27–30.

9. Answer d

In this situation, the patient is stable, as evidenced by being moved from the critical phase of the transplant process, has a high degree of predictability, and has a moderate degree of vulnerability related to the variety of responses related to transfer.

The CNS is demonstrating clinical judgment and caring practices and is acting as a facilitator of learning.

One not so uncommon psychological response to transfer from the intensive care unit is euphoria. The patient may feel that she has beaten the odds and will have a rapid, uncomplicated recovery with the hurdle of surviving surgery and her intensive care stay overcome. By assisting the patient to set realistic goals, the CNS may help the patient avoid developing depression if complications ensue during her continued recovery.

REFERENCES

Curley, M. A. Q. (1998). Patient-Nurse Synergy: Optimizing Patients' Outcomes. *American Journal of Critical Care* 7(1): 64–72.

Glass, C. (1990). *Liver Transplantation.* In B. C. Mims, ed. *Case Studies in Critical Care Nursing* (p. 394). Baltimore, MD: Williams & Wilkins.

Kaplow, R. (2003). AACN Synergy Model for Patient Care: A Framework to Optimize Outcomes. *Critical Care Nurse* 23(Suppl. 1): 27–30.

10. Answer c

In this situation, the CNS is demonstrating clinical judgment and acting as a facilitator of learning.

Elevated peak inspiratory pressures may be due to microvascular thrombi, pulmonary embolism, or acute respiratory distress syndrome (related to thrombosis associated with DIC) or related to interstitial and alveolar edema (related to fibrinolysis of DIC).

REFERENCES

Curley, M. A. Q. (1998). Patient-Nurse Synergy: Optimizing Patients' Outcomes. *American Journal of Critical Care* 7(1): 64–72.

Huddleston, V. B. (1990). Disseminated Intravascular Coagulation. In B. C. Mims, ed. *Case Studies in Critical Care Nursing* (p. 490). Baltimore, MD: Williams & Wilkins.

Kaplow, R. (2003). AACN Synergy Model for Patient Care: A Framework to Optimize Outcomes. *Critical Care Nurse* 23(Suppl. 1): 27–30.

11. Answer d

In this situation, the patient is vulnerable, somewhat predictable because he is exhibiting signs of anxiety, a common response to admission to an intensive care unit.

The CNS in this case is demonstrating clinical judgment and caring practices. Anxiety is one of the most common psychological responses to intensive care admission.

REFERENCES

Curley, M. A. Q. (1998). Patient-Nurse Synergy: Optimizing Patients' Outcomes. *American Journal of Critical Care* 7(1): 64–72.

Kaplow, R. (2003). AACN Synergy Model for Patient Care: A Framework to Optimize Outcomes. *Critical Care Nurse* 23(Suppl. 1): 27–30.

McHugh, L. G., Clark, K. G., and Pierson, D. J. (1992). Psychosocial Aspects of Critical Care: The Patient, the Family, the Staff. Patient Interactions. In D. J. Pierson and R. M. Kacmarek, eds. *Foundations of Respiratory Care* (pp. 1221–1226). New York: Churchill Livingstone.

12. Answer a

In this instance, the nurse is exhibiting clinical judgment. With acute mitral stenosis, less blood is passing through a tight mitral valve. The left ventricular cavity and aorta are often small. Mitral stenosis is associated with a large wave due to increased atrial pressure during atrial systole against a stenotic valve.

REFERENCES

Chan, E. D., Terada, L. S., Kortbeek, J., & Winston, B. W. (2002). *Bedside Critical Care Manual*, 2nd ed. (pp. 85, 162). Philadelphia: Hanley & Belfus.

Curley, M. A. Q. (1998). Patient-Nurse Synergy: Optimizing Patients' Outcomes. *American Journal of Critical Care* 7(1): 64–72.

Kaplow, R. (2003). AACN Synergy Model for Patient Care: A Framework to Optimize Outcomes. *Critical Care Nurse* 23(Suppl. 1): 27–30.

13. Answer d

In this scenario, the CNS is exhibiting clinical judgment and is acting as a facilitator of learning.

The loud apical first sound is due to closure of the stenotic mitral valve. Choice a is incorrect because an S3 gallop is rare because the left ventricle is protected from failure but may be heard. It is caused by blood turbulence in rapid ventricular filling period of early diastole. Choice c is incorrect because an S4 gallop is also rare due to the left ventricle being protected from failure. Choice b is incorrect because mitral stenosis is associated with a rumbling atrial diastolic murmur.

REFERENCES

Curley, M. A. Q. (1998). Patient-Nurse Synergy: Optimizing Patients' Outcomes. *American Journal of Critical Care* 7(1): 64–72.

Kaplow, R. (2003). AACN Synergy Model for Patient Care: A Framework to Optimize Outcomes. *Critical Care Nurse* 23(Suppl. 1): 27–30.

Mims, B. C. (1990). Adult Respiratory Distress Syndrome. In B. C. Mims. *Case Studies in Critical Care Nursing* (p. 174). Baltimore, MD: Williams & Wilkins.

14. Answer b

The patient is vulnerable and is experiencing depersonalization and dehumanization, two types of psychological stress in critical care patients. A trusting relationship between the patient and staff can be established by using the patient's preferred name. Choices a and c work against resolving the feelings of depersonalization and dehumanization. Choice d would be a helpful intervention for sensory deprivation, but will not be effective in the management of the patient's current condition.

REFERENCES

Culver, C. M. (1992). *Ethics at the Bedside*. Hanover, NH: University Press of New England.

Curley, M. A. Q. (1998). Patient-Nurse Synergy: Optimizing Patients' Outcomes. *American Journal of Critical Care* 7(1): 64–72.

Kaplow, R. (2003). AACN Synergy Model for Patient Care: A Framework to Optimize Outcomes. *Critical Care Nurse* 23(Suppl. 1): 27–30.

15. Answer d

In this situation, the patient condition is complex; he is unstable and vulnerable. He has a high level of family participation in care as evidenced by the wife visiting and caring about the patient and son. Choice a is an incorrect belief. Choice b is incorrect because refusal to allow the child to visit may lead the imagination to be worse than reality. Choice c would not promote the best outcome for the patient and family. Choice d is correct because it will enhance participation in care and increase family coping with the hospitalization. The nurse, in this instance, is acting as a moral advocate for the patient and family.

REFERENCES

Culver, C. M. (1992). *Ethics at the Bedside*. Hanover, NH: University Press of New England.
Curley, M. A. Q. (1998). Patient-Nurse Synergy: Optimizing Patients' Outcomes. *American Journal of Critical Care* 7(1): 64–72.
Kaplow, R. (2003). AACN Synergy Model for Patient Care: A Framework to Optimize Outcomes. *Critical Care Nurse* 23(Suppl. 1): 27–30.

16. Answer d

The patient and family are vulnerable at this time. The patient is unstable. Choice a is incorrect because it is not clear what dysfunction, if any, the patient has incurred as a result of the cardiopulmonary arrest. This intervention will not address the wife's concerns. Choice b is incorrect because the patient should be encouraged to enroll in these groups upon discharge from the ICU and these interventions will not help the wife with her concerns. Choice c is incorrect because providing written materials about cardiopulmonary resuscitation will not adequately equip the wife to perform rescue techniques if she is witness to another arrest. It also is not clear what her apprehension is related to. Lack of knowledge may not be the etiology of her concerns. Further exploration of the wife's concerns is indicated in this situation. This is best reflected in Choice d.

REFERENCES

Culver, C. M. (1992). *Ethics at the Bedside*. Hanover, NH: University Press of New England.
Curley, M. A. Q. (1998). Patient-Nurse Synergy: Optimizing Patients' Outcomes. *American Journal of Critical Care* 7(1): 64–72.
Kaplow, R. (2003). AACN Synergy Model for Patient Care: A Framework to Optimize Outcomes. *Critical Care Nurse* 23(Suppl. 1): 27–30.

17. Answer c

In this instance, the CNS is exhibiting clinical judgment and is acting as a facilitator of learning. Overdrive pacing is the use of pacemaker impulses to regulate heart rate and rhythm. Pacing the heart at a faster rate than the patient's current heart rate may interrupt the tachycardia and allow the SA node to regain control of the heart. Hence, in order for overdrive pacing to be effective, the rate on the pacemaker must be set at a rate higher than the patient's current heart rate.

REFERENCES

Curley, M. A. Q. (1998). Patient-Nurse Synergy: Optimizing Patients' Outcomes. *American Journal of Critical Care* 7(1): 64–72.

DelMonte, L., and Gamrath, B. (1996). *Noninvasive Pacing. What You Should Know*, 2nd ed. Redmond, WA: Physio-Control Corporation.

Kaplow, R. (2003). AACN Synergy Model for Patient Care: A Framework to Optimize Outcomes. *Critical Care Nurse* 23(Suppl. 1): 27–30.

18. Answer b

In this instance, the CNS is exhibiting clinical judgment and is acting as a facilitator of learning. If the aorta is weak from an aneurysm, placement of an intraaortic balloon pump could perforate the aorta. This can result in patient death.

REFERENCES

Curley, M. A. Q. (1998). Patient-Nurse Synergy: Optimizing Patients' Outcomes. *American Journal of Critical Care* 7(1): 64–72.

Gilworth, D. L. (1990). Cardiac Case Study. In B. C. Mims, ed. *Case Studies in Critical Care Nursing* (p. 41). Baltimore, MD: Williams & Wilkins.

Kaplow, R. (2003). AACN Synergy Model for Patient Care: A Framework to Optimize Outcomes. *Critical Care Nurse* 23(Suppl. 1): 27–30.

19. Answer a

In this instance, the CNS is exhibiting clinical judgment. Due to the lack of perfusion distal to the occlusion, muscle ischemia and cell death occur. This causes liberation of potassium, magnesium, and lactic acidosis. Upon reperfusion, these substances are released into the systemic circulation. The lactic acidosis results in hyperkalemia related to the patient being acidotic. Sodium bicarbonate administration causes pH and potassium to return to within normal limits.

REFERENCES

Curley, M. A. Q. (1998). Patient-Nurse Synergy: Optimizing Patients' Outcomes. *American Journal of Critical Care* 7(1): 64–72.

Huddleston, V. B. (1990). Femoral Popliteal Bypass. In B. C. Mims, ed. *Case Studies in Critical Care Nursing* (p. 72). Baltimore, MD: Williams & Wilkins.

Kaplow, R. (2003). AACN Synergy Model for Patient Care: A Framework to Optimize Outcomes. *Critical Care Nurse* 23(Suppl. 1): 27–30.

20. Answer c

In this situation, the CNS is acting as a facilitator of learning, advocate and moral agent, and is exhibiting caring practices and clinical judgment. Decisions to withhold, withdraw, or continue life-sustaining treatment may be made by the patient, the patient's surrogate, or by the patient's physician. The decisions that are made by patients reflect their right to approve or refuse any treatment modality including those that sustain life. For patients who lack decision-making capacity, either due to an underlying disease or use of sedating agents, surrogates may make decisions for the patient using a "best interests" perspective. When a patient lacks decision-making capacity and surrogates are not available, the patient's physician may make decisions about the patient's therapies based on that same principle of "best interest."

REFERENCES

Curley, M. A. Q. (1998). Patient-Nurse Synergy: Optimizing Patients' Outcomes. *American Journal of Critical Care* 7(1): 64–72.

Kaplow, R. (2003). AACN Synergy Model for Patient Care: A Framework to Optimize Outcomes. *Critical Care Nurse* 23(Suppl. 1): 27–30.

Kapp, M. B. (2001). Legal Liability Anxieties in the ICU. In J. R. Curtis and G. D. Rubemfeld, (Eds.) *Managing Death in the ICU: The Transition from Cure to Comfort*. New York: Oxford University Press.

Luce, J. M., & Alpers, A. (2000). Legal Aspects of Withholding and Withdrawing Life Support from Critically Ill Patients in the United States and Providing Palliative Care to Them. *American Journal of Respiratory Critical Care Medicine* 162: 2029–2032.

21. Answer c

In this situation, the CNS is acting as an advocate and moral agent and is exhibiting caring practices and clinical judgment. When patients lack decision-making capacity and surrogates are not available, decisions are often made by the patient's physician, usually acting in collaboration with clinical colleagues and, possibly, the hospital ethics committee. Physicians use the "best interest" standard when deciding to withhold or withdraw support for patients if they deem treatment is "futile" and is, therefore, not in the patient's best interest. The American Medical Association has argued that "physicians are not ethically obligated to deliver care that, in their best professional judgment, will not have a reasonable chance of benefiting their patients." Choices a, b, and d may not advocate for the patient's "best interest."

REFERENCES

American Medical Association Council on Ethics and Judicial Affairs. (1997). *Code of Medical Ethics: Current Opinions and Annotations.* Chicago, IL: American Medical Association.

Curley, M. A. Q. (1998). Patient-Nurse Synergy: Optimizing Patients' Outcomes. *American Journal of Critical Care* 7(1): 64–72.

Kaplow, R. (2003). AACN Synergy Model for Patient Care: A Framework to Optimize Outcomes. *Critical Care Nurse* 23(Suppl. 1): 27–30.

Luce, J. M. (2002). Three Patients Who Asked that Life Support Be Withheld or Withdrawn in the Surgical Intensive Care Unit. *Critical Care Medicine* 30: 775–780.

22. Answer c

In this situation, the CNS is acting as an advocate and moral agent and is exhibiting caring practices, clinical judgment, and clinical inquiry. Adherence to infection control practices is paramount in order to prevent the spread of infection from one patient to another. By asking the physician to step outside and don the appropriate isolation attire, the CNS is exhibiting knowledge of infection control practices. The CNS might also act as a facilitator of learning if the lack of compliance with infection control practices by the physician was related to a knowledge deficit.

REFERENCES

Curley, M. A. Q. (1998). Patient-Nurse Synergy: Optimizing Patients' Outcomes. *American Journal of Critical Car,* 7(1): 64–72.

Kaplow, R. (2003). AACN Synergy Model for Patient Care: A Framework to Optimize Outcomes. *Critical Care Nurse* 23(Suppl. 1): 27–30.

23. Answer b

In this situation, the nurse is exhibiting caring practices and is acting as an advocate and moral agent for the family. The patient described in the scenario is unstable, has high levels of complexity and vulnerability, and low abilities for decision making and participation in care.

When a patient is hospitalized, the waiting room of the intensive care unit often becomes a 24-hour home for the families. After a few days, it is not uncommon for families to have feelings of helplessness and lack of control. The advanced practice nurse can help the family deal with these feelings of helplessness of lack of control by working to identify tasks into which their energies can be usefully channeled.

Families need clear information about the elements of treatment, the rationales for the treatments, and that these may change over time. The CNS should emphasize that the staff caring for the patient will continue to be honest and that the staff can understand how difficult it is for the family to deal with the continual anxiety of an uncertain prognosis. Family conferences offer another way to facilitate communication and reduce conflict between staff and family and among family members. Conferences also provide a good opportunity for staff to assess the family members' coping abilities.

REFERENCES

Curley, M. A. Q. (1998). Patient-Nurse Synergy: Optimizing Patients' Outcomes. *American Journal of Critical Care* 7(1): 64–72.

Kaplow, R. (2003). AACN Synergy Model for Patient Care: A Framework to Optimize Outcomes. *Critical Care Nurse* 23(Suppl. 1): 27–30.

McHugh, L. G., Clark, K. G., and Pierson, D. J. (1992). Psychosocial Aspects of Critical Care: The Patient, the Family, the Staff. Patient Interactions. In D.J. Pierson and R. M. Kacmarek, eds. *Foundations of Respiratory Care* (pp. 1221–1226). New York: Churchill Livingstone.

24. Answer b

In this situation, the CNS is exhibiting clinical judgment, caring practices, clinical inquiry, and facilitator of learning. In this situation, the CNS is utilizing research findings, demonstrating ability in clinical inquiry, and creating a practice change. By assisting the nurse to turn the patient on the inappropriate side (choice a) or assisting the nurse with chest physiotherapy and postural drainage on the incorrect side (choice d), optimal patient outcomes would likely not occur. Leaving research articles (choice c) will eventually help to teach the nurse the evidence to support positioning the patient with the "good lung down," but will not address the immediate issue. In patients with unilateral lung disease, positioning the "good lung down" increases oxygenation by improving ventilation: perfusion (V/Q) matching due to gravitational effects on blood flow.

REFERENCES

Bridges, E. J. (2001). Ask the Experts. *Critical Care Nurse,* 21(6): 66–68.

Curley, M. A. Q. (1998). Patient-Nurse Synergy: Optimizing Patients' Outcomes. *American Journal of Critical Care* 7(1): 64–72.

Kaplow, R. (2003). AACN Synergy Model for Patient Care: A Framework to Optimize Outcomes. *Critical Care Nurse* 23(Suppl. 1): 27–30.

25. Answer d

In this situation, the CNS is exhibiting clinical inquiry, caring practices, and is acting as an advocate and moral agent on behalf of the patient and family.

Several categories of needs of a patient's family in the ICU have been identified in research studies. These needs include being in attendance with the patient, receiving information on the condition of the patient, feeling useful, having the opportunity to express feelings about the situation, and receiving emotional support. The CNS, by utilizing research findings and creating a practice change, is exhibiting ability in clinical inquiry. By representing concerns of the family, the CNS is acting as an advocate to help resolve a concern in the clinical setting. The CNS is attempting to create a compassionate, supportive, and therapeutic environment for the family (caring practices), trying to prevent unnecessary suffering.

REFERENCES

Curley, M. A. Q. (1998). Patient-Nurse Synergy: Optimizing Patients' Outcomes. *American Journal of Critical Care* 7(1): 64–72.

Kaplow, R. (2003). AACN Synergy Model for Patient Care: A Framework to Optimize Outcomes. *Critical Care Nurs,* 23(Suppl. 1): 27–30.

McHugh, L. G., Clark, K. G., and Pierson, D. J. (1992). Psychosocial Aspects of Critical Care: The Patient, the Family, the Staff. Patient Interactions. In D. J. Pierson and R. M. Kacmarek, eds. *Foundations of Respiratory Care* (pp. 1221–1236). New York: Churchill Livingstone.

CHAPTER 23

THE CARE OF THE ACUTE AND CRITICALLY ILL ADULT PATIENT IN THE PROGRESSIVE CARE UNIT SAMPLE QUESTIONS

Marthe J. Moseley, PhD, RN, CCRN, CCNS

INTRODUCTION

The following questions have been developed to provide examples of questions that integrate the patient and nurse characteristics of the AACN Synergy Model. The questions in this chapter focus on the acute and critically ill adult patient in the progressive care unit (PCU) environment. An annotated answer key based on the AACN Synergy Model is at the end of the set of questions to provide rationale for the correct choice and for why the other choices are not the best answer.

1. A patient with high blood pressure is being monitored for response to antihypertensive therapy. The patient's family asks if they can spend time with the patient and wonder if visiting him or holding the patient's hand would be acceptable. The best response from the nurse would be to say:
   a. "No, because further stimulation may compound his already hypertensive condition."
   b. "Yes, maybe your presence at the bedside will help him relax."
   c. "No, because it interferes with the multiple blood pressure checks necessary to determine appropriate response to medical interventions."
   d. "Yes, and I will continue to assess his response."

2. The caretaker of an acutely ill progressive care patient appears uncertain and explains, "I feel like I am unable to support my friend in any way." Appropriate nursing interventions would include:
   a. Confirming the report and offering solutions to problems identified by the caretaker.
   b. Encouraging the support of the other family members and eliciting their help to make crucial choices in the health care plan.

    c. Providing reassurance and stating that visiting is not always necessary by the caretaker because nursing care is being provided.

    d. Validating the statement with the caretaker and identifying and reinforcing current support systems.

3. A patient is being transferred from the ICU to the PCU after an ICU stay of 3 months. The family is anxious and pensive. Which of the following nursing interventions do patients' family members perceive as a caring behavior?

    a. Supplying detailed explanations of PCU equipment and unit specific policies.

    b. Orienting the family to the progressive care environment.

    c. Consulting with the PCU physicians for provision of transfer information.

    d. Organizing family members to participate in patient care and visitation.

4. A non-English speaking patient is admitted to the PCU and is unable to communicate with the health care team. When coordinating care with the family of this patient, the most effective means of communicating with the non-English speaking family would be by utilizing:

    a. Translation services

    b. A bilingual daughter to interpret

    c. Ancillary staff for explanation

    d. A communication board

5. A postoperative patient with a history of sleep apnea reports that his surgical pain is a 7 on a scale of 0 to 10. The charge nurse reports that male surgical patients tend to have a lower tolerance for any level of pain. The best response from the nurse would be:

    a. "This patient has lower pain tolerance."

    b. "High-risk postsurgery patients are at risk for respiratory depression and thus need to have some pain."

    c. "Abdominal surgery produces the most intense pain and should always be treated whenever the health care provider feels that the patient is in acute pain."

    d. "Pain is experienced differently by each patient."

6. A nurse is facilitating diabetic teaching with a patient who is visually challenged. The most useful teaching strategy would be to:

    a. Provide a simplified description of the complete diabetes program to the patient.

    b. Show an educational videotape to the patient's family.

    c. Provide verbal descriptions of diabetes care to the patient.

    d. Eliminate use of the food models during the food-planning session.

7. A 40-year-old patient admitted for rule out myocardial infarction has a negative set of cardiac enzymes from the first lab draw. The patient appears withdrawn and is not interested in being involved in any aspect of care. To approach this issue with the patient, the most appropriate statement by the nurse might be:

a. "How are you with your heart disease?"
b. "Would you like to talk about the care you are getting?"
c. "Do you want to involve your family in your care at this time?"
d. "May I teach you about how to make healthy food choices?"

8. A PCU patient who was admitted from the ED has no pulse or respirations. What action is probably the most essential responsibility of the nurse after a code has been called?
   a. Intubating the patient and managing the airway.
   b. Summarizing applicable history including diagnostic results for the health care team.
   c. Starting an intravenous line for administration of medications.
   d. Providing the team leader an update on physiological events prior to the code.

9. A patient has a wound infection with dressing changes ordered twice a day. Several family members think that the patient is in great pain during dressing changes and believe that therapeutic touch would help with pain management. The hospital does not have staff who practice therapeutic touch, but the family has contacted a group of providers for this therapy. Hospital policy allows visitation only by family members. Which of the following would be the most important perspective about the consideration of this therapy?
   a. Alternative methods have correlated with enhancements in pharmacologic effects.
   b. No evidence exists to support the value of therapeutic touch in pain management.
   c. Complementary therapies are not generally acceptable in a PCU setting given the critical nature of the patients.
   d. Coordinate a team conference with the family members to explain the rationale for hospital visitation policies.

10. A large family assembly has gathered in the PCU team conference room. They have been praying together throughout the day as the health of their family member declines. One of the patient's siblings is now using incense. The interaction between family members has become louder as the patient's health worsens. The family members of the other patients in the PCU have requested to move this family to another area. The most appropriate action of the nurse should be to:
    a. Meet with the family to establish a mutual means for meeting their needs.
    b. Notify the contact person in the large family that religious ceremonies involving groups of people are scheduled in the hospital chapel.
    c. Remove the incense from the conference room and inform the family of the fire hazard policy.
    d. Reassure the other families that the hospital staff will manage the situation.

11. A patient is in the PCU with end-stage cardiomyopathy. Having established a relationship with the patient and family after multiple hospital admissions, the patient has now decided to stop all aggressive treatment and desires to be placed in hospice. After meeting the physical needs of the patient, the nurse notes that the patient appears restless. The most appropriate intervention by the nurse is to:
    a. Sedate the patient to lessen anxiety.
    b. Defer any other physical care until the patient is calm.
    c. Use touch to soothe the patient thereby promoting relaxation.
    d. Give approval for family members to constantly stay with the patient.

12. A family member asks if children are permitted to visit the patient in the PCU. The children are members of the family but have never been in a hospital before. The nurse may inform the family member to:
    a. Persuade the children to visit alone having visits spaced through the day so as to not tire the patient.
    b. Describe the hospital environment to the children, offering them pictures to clarify any questions.
    c. Tell the children that their family member might look very sick but probably will not die.
    d. Determine the wishes of the children and see if they want to visit their family member.

13. A previously disruptive family member telephones the nurse in the PCU seeking permission to visit a patient after their work shift ends near midnight. To address this request, the nurse's best response would be to:
    a. Quote the visitation policy emphasizing that visits need to occur at the scheduled time.
    b. Inquire about visitation before the work shift starts and clear this request with the nurse manager's approval.
    c. Not allow the visit, because the patient, along with the other patients, will be sleeping.
    d. Permit visitation as requested after setting behavioral limits.

14. A patient with a permanent tracheostomy has begun the discharge process. The spouse has asked questions about how to keep the airway open, has asked about eating pureed foods, and has concerns about home oxygen use and delivery schedules as well as wondering if someone is to come into the home at night time when the spouse would be sleeping. The best response by the nurse would be:
    a. "The ear, nose, and throat nurse specialist will come and practice suctioning with you."
    b. "We can begin with your main concern."
    c. "We can have dietary service tell you which blender is best for pureed foods."
    d. "Oxygen delivery should not be a problem."

15. During rounds in the PCU, one of the consulting service physicians is asked by the patient if cancer was found. Knowing that the family members of the patient do not want any information given to the patient regarding the diagnosis, what would be the best reply by the nurse when the physician looks to him for a response?
    a. "Your primary care physician will be notified that you have questions."
    b. "Your condition will be discussed and we will return to tell you."
    c. "We do not have all of the diagnostic test results back at this time."
    d. "We will bring your family in and discuss this with you."

16. A patient who had a CABG 3 months ago is due to be admitted with postoperative complications including sternal wound infection. In addition, the patient is a diabetic. The PCU is full, and the only other hospital bed is in the medical patient care setting. The nurse should *first*:
    a. Collaborate with the physician on triage of the current patients.
    b. Arrange for the patient with multiple problems to be transferred to the other unit.
    c. Transfer any patient with DNR orders to the medicine unit.
    d. Hold the patient with the sternal wound infection in the emergency room.

17. A patient requiring complex care has been in the PCU for many months. The family members have been continually demanding and now the relationship between the family of the patient and PCU health team members has become strained. The best response by the nurse should be to:
    a. Discuss the situation with the medical team.
    b. Propose that the family verbalize their concerns with the nurse manager.
    c. Rotate assignments every day among staff members to decrease stress.
    d. Coordinate a patient care conference to include the family.

18. A patient in the PCU has family members who are expressing a desire to be more involved in the actual care for the patient. The most appropriate response would be to:
    a. Encourage the family to assist with physical care routines.
    b. Explain that the complex care requires special training.
    c. Tell the family that the patient is not aware of who the caregivers are.
    d. Request the family to observe patient care procedures to facilitate discharge care.

19. When planning care for a PCU patient in a highly catabolic state or stressed state, the nurse should initially consult which of the following?
    a. Gastroenterologist
    b. Physical therapist
    c. Registered dietician
    d. Respiratory therapist

20. An education session has been planned with the family members of a PCU patient. The nurse's initial teaching approach is to understand that the family:
    a. Is usually ready to be taught at any time because they are willing to aid in giving care.
    b. Learns best if they perceive a need to learn.
    c. Learns optimally if shown a complicated procedure all at one time.
    d. Wants limited responsibility for dimensions of physical care.

21. When gathering supplies to perform endotracheal suctioning, a peer assists by adding normal saline vials to the gathered equipment. The peer justifies saline instillation because it loosens secretions. The most appropriate response would be to:
    a. Ensure in-line ventilator humidification on the inhalation circuit.
    b. Increase the patient's IV fluid intake to provide adequate hydration.
    c. Discuss with the peer the research contraindicating this practice.
    d. Report the peer's actions to the nurse manager.

22. To determine how the family is doing in response to a patient's long-term illness, the most appropriate response by the nurse is to ask:
    a. "Do you know what is going on?"
    b. "Can I do something for you?"
    c. "What is your understanding of the situation?"
    d. "Do you have any questions of me?"

23. A PCU patient is weak and unable to participate in ADLs. Attempts by the nurse to initiate care result in verbal criticism from the patient's family member. In continuing the plan of care, the most beneficial intervention would include:
    a. Rotating ADL care assignments for the patient.
    b. Scheduling a conference with the patient, family member, and staff.
    c. Obtaining a psychiatric consultation for the family member.
    d. Limitation of visitation to non-ADL times of the day.

24. A plan to teach wound care to the son of a patient has been implemented. The son has not been successful in demonstrating the skill. Which intervention would be most appropriate next step?
    a. Provide coaching and the opportunity to repeat the skill.
    b. Ask the wound care specialist to consult on the teaching.
    c. Eliminate dressing changes from the procedure the son will perform.
    d. Provide written step-by-step instructions for the son.

25. The family has not left the bedside of their loved one since admission 5 days ago. The patient's family verbally expresses anger and does not seem to understand basic information provided by the health care team. Which of the following interventions should be utilized first?
    a. Clarify the family's perception of the problem.
    b. Teach the family how to assist with the easy procedures.
    c. Encourage open visitation by the family.
    d. Provide consistent updates on the patient's condition.

ANSWER KEY TO THE CARE OF THE ACUTE AND CRITICALLY ILL
ADULT PATIENT IN THE PCU SAMPLE QUESTIONS WITH RATIONALES

1. Answer d

Because this patient is moderately vulnerable, the patient is somewhat susceptible to actual or potential stressors that may adversely affect the patient's outcome. In addition, the patient would be highly complex, due to the intricate entanglement of two or more systems. Given the patient's complexity and vulnerability, choices a, b, and c would not be correct because they do not consider the combination of the patient's characteristics according to the Synergy Model. The best response in this scenario is to ensure that the needs of the patient and family member are met in a caring environment. Accomplishing this while synthesizing and interpreting the blood pressure changes in response to the therapy is the best approach.

REFERENCES

Curley, M. A.Q. (1998). Patient-Nurse Synergy: Optimizing Patients' Outcomes. *American Journal of Critical Care* 7(1): 64–72.
Collopy, K. S. (1999). The Synergy Model in Practice: Advanced Practice Nurses Guiding Families Through Systems. *Critical Care Nurse* 19(5): 80–5.

2. Answer d

The caretaker is a support system of the patient. At this present time, the capacity to participate in care is less than optimal. In addition, the family unit is moderately complex due to the entanglement of two or more systems. The best response in this situation is to validate what the caretaker is saying and to spend some time in identifying the presence of support systems other than the caretaker. Working with the caretaker to identify solutions rather than offering solutions is the better approach. It is unknown whether there are other support systems, thus engaging use of them would not be the best response at this time. In addition, having the caretaker not visit is not a realistic expectation in terms of taking positive steps toward resolution of the problem itself.

REFERENCES

Curley, M. A.Q. (1998). Patient-Nurse Synergy: Optimizing Patients' Outcomes. *American Journal of Critical Care* 7(1): 64–72.
Collopy, K. S. (1999). The Synergy Model in Practice: Advanced Practice Nurses Guiding Families Through Systems. *Critical Care Nurse* 19(5): 80–5.

3. Answer b

The patient and family at this moment of transfer would be classified as highly vulnerable. The patient has had an ICU stay of 3 months and their actual or potential stressors may definitely affect the patient's outcome. The willingness to participate in care is moderate because this is a new care environment. In addition, the participation in decision making is also moderate, because input and advice from others will be needed in the new care environment. Therefore, the caring behavior would be identified as one, which showed the facilitation or implementation of a process to ensure that the needs of the patient and family are met to navigate along this time of transition. The caring behavior would be to orient the family to the new environment. Supplying detailed explanations, consulting with the physicians, and organizing family members would not be a characteristic definition within caring practices.

REFERENCES

Curley, M. A.Q. (1998). Patient-Nurse Synergy: Optimizing Patients' Outcomes. *American Journal of Critical Care* 7(1): 64–72.
Mullen, J. E. (2002). The Synergy Model in Practice: The Synergy Model as a Framework for Nursing Rounds. *Critical Care Nurse* 22(6): 66–79.

4. Answer a

The patient and family members who do not speak the primary language of the care environment are considered fragile in terms of vulnerability. In addition, the availability of resources may be somewhat limited, in terms of having access to information. Given these considerations, the nursing characteristics that are most needed at this time include response to diversity to tailor the delivery of care to meet the needs of the patient and systems thinking to anticipate consequences of changes in systems and develop proactive strategies for this patient and family. The effective means of communication is through translation services. Relying on the daughter, ancillary staff, or a communication board is not considered the most effective means of communication.

REFERENCES

Curley, M. A.Q. (1998). Patient-Nurse Synergy: Optimizing Patients' Outcomes. *American Journal of Critical Care* 7(1): 64–72.
Mullen, J. E. (2002). The Synergy Model in Practice: The Synergy Model as a Framework for Nursing Rounds. *Critical Care Nurse* 22(6): 66–79.

5. Answer d

This patient admitted postoperative for sleep apnea would be considered highly complex and minimally stable given the potential for airway management issues. Most patients, if they are in the hospital at this point, have an alteration in maintaining an adequate airway. Compounded by the need for adequate pain management, this patient presents as complex in terms of understanding the need to keep the pain level tolerable and continue to optimize gas exchange. The nurse characteristics that fit the needs of the patient at this time include clinical judgment skills to make complex decisions based on the patient's diagnosis and pain, and clinical inquiry to teach about the research recommendations, and the adoption of them into clinical practice. Thus the best response would be choice d. Choices a, b, and c do not incorporate research recommendations.

REFERENCES

Curley, M. A.Q. (1998). Patient-Nurse Synergy: Optimizing Patients' Outcomes. *American Journal of Critical Care* 7(1): 64–72.
Collopy, K. S. (1999). The Synergy Model in Practice: Advanced Practice Nurses Guiding Families Through Systems. *Critical Care Nurse* 19(5): 80–5.

6. Answer c

In facilitating learning for this patient, resource availability is a high need. Given the visual challenges, the nurse must locate supportive resources that will optimize learning. The predictability of this patient could be moderately wavering. Ongoing reassessment of each step of the teaching process is a must to ensure that the patient understands each section of the teaching sessions. In addition, sessions should be clustered into an adequate number of sessions to ensure that the patient has met the learning plan and the nurse has met the patient's needs.

REFERENCES

Curley, M. A.Q. (1998). Patient-Nurse Synergy: Optimizing Patients' Outcomes. *American Journal of Critical Care* 7(1): 64–72.
Collopy, K. S. (1999). The Synergy Model in Practice: Advanced Practice Nurses Guiding Families Through Systems. *Critical Care Nurse* 19(5): 80–5.

7. Answer a

This patient is unwilling to participate in care. It is important that when engaging in conversation with a patient that open-ended questioning is used to elicit more than a yes or no response. Thus, the choices of b, c, or d would not promote ongoing discussion and thus would not be the best choice. The best nurse characteristic would be that of caring practice to ensure that the needs of the patient are met in terms of healing and powerlessness. To identify the needs of the patient, the nurse must promote open communication.

REFERENCES

Curley, M. A.Q. (1998). Patient-Nurse Synergy: Optimizing Patients' Outcomes. *American Journal of Critical Care* 7(1): 64–72.

Collopy, K. S. (1999). The Synergy Model in Practice: Advanced Practice Nurses Guiding Families Through Systems. *Critical Care Nurse,* 19(5): 80–5.

8. Answer d

Given the emergent situation in which the patient is highly vulnerable, minimally stable, and highly complex, in order to determine the outcome of the patient, the best response of the nurse following the initiation of the code team is to provide an update on the clinical events that happened prior to the code. The nurse must collaborate with the code team to provide vital information to optimize patient recovery. Choices a and c are interventions that are typically provided by a member of the code team. Choice b is not relevant at this time because it asked for a history including diagnostic results.

REFERENCES

Annis, T. D. (2002). The Synergy Model in Practice: The Interdisciplinary Team Across the Continuum of Care. *Critical Care Nurse* 22(5): 76–79.

Curley, M. A.Q. (1998). Patient-Nurse Synergy: Optimizing Patients' Outcomes. *American Journal of Critical Care* 7(1): 64–72.

Collopy, K. S. (1999). Advanced Practice Nurses Guiding Families Through Systems. *Critical Care Nurse* 19(5).

9. Answer a

This patient and the family system would best be categorized as highly complex and dynamic. There is an intricate entanglement of two or more systems. Although the hospital policy only allows for family visitation, making available the resources that the family is requesting needs to be considered because alternative methods of therapy have been correlated with patient benefit. The nurse characteristics of clinical judgment, clinical inquiry, and response to diversity are needed to make decisions based on this complex case. Choices b and c are not the best responses because they do not incorporate current research results. Choice d is not the best response because a team conference is not the place to explain policies.

REFERENCES

Curley, M. A.Q. (1998). Patient-Nurse Synergy: Optimizing Patients' Outcomes. *American Journal of Critical Care* 7(1): 64–72.

Collopy, K. S. (1999). The Synergy Model in Practice: Advanced Practice Nurses Guiding Families Through Systems. *Critical Care Nurse* 19(5):80–5.

10. Answer a

As this patient's health is worsening, the stability of the patient would be considered as minimal given the high risk of death. In addition, the complexity of the patient/family dynamics is high. To provide for the patient/family unit as a whole, given the resources that exist in this hospital setting, the best response would be to gather the family to establish a means to meet the needs. This intervention will promote dialogue with the family unit. The nurse characteristics that are most needed at this time are that of the combination of response to diversity and clinical judgment. Integrating the protocols and complex care decisions within the framework of the family wishes leads to choosing the most appropriate response as a.

REFERENCES

Curley, M. A.Q. (1998). Patient-Nurse Synergy: Optimizing Patients' Outcomes. *American Journal of Critical Care* 7(1): 64–72.

Collopy, K. S. (1999). The Synergy Model in Practice: Advanced Practice Nurses Guiding Families Through Systems. *Critical Care Nurse* 19(5): 80–5.

11. Answer c

An assessment of this patient is that the patient is highly vulnerable and ready to die. In addition, the stability and resiliency of the patient is minimal. The nursing characteristics most needed at this time include a combination of clinical judgment, advocacy/moral agency, and caring practices. The most appropriate intervention by the nurse would be to ensure that more than physical care is provided; thus, choice c would be the best response. Sedating the patient does not meet the psychological needs of the patient. Deferring care will not meet the psychological need. Family visitation, although appropriate, may not meet the need at this time, because the patient is restless.

REFERENCES

Curley, M. A.Q. (1998). Patient-Nurse Synergy: Optimizing Patients' Outcomes. *American Journal of Critical Care* 7(1): 64–72.

Hardin, S., & Hussey, L. (2003). AACN Synergy Model for Patient Care: Case Study of a CHF Patient. *Critical Care Nurse* 23(1): 73–76.

Collopy, K. S. (1999). The Synergy Model in Practice: Advanced Practice Nurses Guiding Families Through Systems. *Critical Care Nurse* 19(5): 80–5.

12. Answer d

The request to include children into the hospital environment adds to the complexity of patient/family dynamics. In addition, not knowing if the system has resources available such as having a child life specialist to assess the readiness of the children, the best response would be to determine the wishes of the children. The nurse characteristics of systems thinking, clinical judgment, and facilitator of learning would best meet the needs at this time. Further assessment of the wishes of the children is the first step of these choices that needs to be determined before a plan can be further developed to include visitation by the children.

REFERENCES

Curley, M. A.Q. (1998). Patient-Nurse Synergy: Optimizing Patients' Outcomes. *American Journal of Critical Care* 7(1): 64–72.

Collopy, K. S. (1999). The Synergy Model in Practice: Advanced Practice Nurses Guiding Families Through Systems. *Critical Care Nurse* 19(5): 80–5.

13. Answer d

Given the history of disruptive behavior, the complexity of the patient/family dynamic would be considered high. Coupling advocacy and moral agency with caring practices enables the nurse to establish an environment to promote the rights of the patients and their families yet ensure safe passage. Behavioral limit setting is key for safe passage of the patient. The other three choices do not encourage incorporating the wishes of the family member and thus would not be the best responses.

REFERENCES

Curley, M. A.Q. (1998). Patient-Nurse Synergy: Optimizing Patients' Outcomes. *American Journal of Critical Care* 7(1): 64–72.

Collopy, K. S. (1999). The Synergy Model in Practice: Advanced Practice Nurses Guiding Families Through Systems. *Critical Care Nurse* 19(5): 80–5.

14. Answer b

Given the number of concerns voiced by the spouse of the patient, one can identify that the actual or potential stressors that may adversely affect the patient's outcome would be identified as high. In addition, the complexity of the care requirements would also be considered high. It is important that the nurse characteristics of facilitator of learning and clinical inquiry combine to determine the highest priority at the current time. Choice b encourages the priority setting be made by the family member. Choices a, c, and d may not encourage further discussion to ensure meeting the family members' needs.

REFERENCES

Curley, M. A.Q. (1998). Patient-Nurse Synergy: Optimizing Patients' Outcomes. *American Journal of Critical Care* 7(1): 64–72.

Collopy, K. S. (1999). The Synergy Model in Practice: Advanced Practice Nurses Guiding Families Through Systems. *Critical Care Nurse* 19(5): 80–5.

15. Answer d

This patient would be classified as highly vulnerable and minimally stable due to a recent diagnosis. In addition, given the complexity of the family situation, there is an intricate and very complex dynamic within the patient and family system. The nurse characteristics of advocacy and moral agency along with response to diversity promotes establishment of an environment that encourages ethical decision making yet tailors the delivery of care to meet the needs and strengths of the patient, family, and staff. This complex issue requires that the patient, family, and staff are present to hear the information given. Choices a, b, and c do not address the question and leave the ethical issue open. Choice d ensures that all of the team members and family will be present as the patient is informed of the response to his question.

REFERENCES

Curley, M. A.Q. (1998). Patient-Nurse Synergy: Optimizing Patients' Outcomes. *American Journal of Critical Care* 7(1): 64–72.
Collopy, K. S. (1999). The Synergy Model in Practice: Advanced Practice Nurses Guiding Families Through Systems. *Critical Care Nurse* 19(5): 80–5.

16. Answer a

This patient is highly complex given the existence of the sternal wound infection and the coexisting diagnosis of diabetes. The nurse characteristics needed at this time include clinical judgment, systems thinking, and collaboration. The decision to transfer into and out of the unit must be made in collaboration with the head physician of the PCU. Given the complexity of the patient care requirements, the nurse should first concur with the physician, thus the choices of b, c, and d are not the most appropriate responses.

REFERENCES

Curley, M. A.Q. (1998). Patient-Nurse Synergy: Optimizing Patients' Outcomes. *American Journal of Critical Care* 7(1): 64–72.
Ecklund, M. M., and Stamps, D. C. (2002). The Synergy Model in Practice: Promoting Synergy in Progressive Care. *Critical Care Nurse* 22(4): 60–66.
Collopy, K. S. (1999). The Synergy Model in Practice: Advanced practice nurses guiding families through systems. *Critical Care Nurse* 19(5): 80–5.

17. Answer d

This patient is highly complex. Given the length of stay over many months, resiliency is at a minimum. In order to optimize the ability of the family to participate in care and in decision making, it is imperative that input and advice from, others is needed given the strained situation. The nurse characteristics most needed at this time include collaboration and caring practices. Leading the team to focus on the issues involving the family to ensure their needs are met will aid in optimizing the patient/family outcomes. Choice d is the best response of the nurse. Choices a, b, and c will not resolve the issue of the strained relationship.

REFERENCES

Annis, T. D. (2002). The Synergy Model in Practice: The Interdisciplinary Team Across the Continuum of Care. *Critical Care Nurse* 22(5): 76–79.
Curley, M. A.Q. (1998). Patient-Nurse Synergy: Optimizing Patients' Outcomes. *American Journal of Critical Care* 7(1): 64–72.
Collopy, K. S. (1999). The Synergy Model in Practice: Advanced practice nurses guiding families through systems. *Critical Care Nurse* 19(5).

18. Answer a

Upon making the assessment that the family desires to participate in care to a full level, the nurse should make every opportunity available to meet this request. Using clinical judgment and the facilitator of learning characteristics, the nurse would best meet the needs of the patient's family by encouraging assistance. Choices b, c, and d do not include involvement which is what is requested; thus, choice a would be the best response.

REFERENCES

Curley, M. A.Q. (1998). Patient-Nurse Synergy: Optimizing Patients' Outcomes. *American Journal of Critical Care* 7(1): 64–72.
Mullen, J. E. (2002). The Synergy Model in Practice: The Synergy Model as a Framework for Nursing Rounds. *Critical Care Nurse* 22(6): 66–79.

19. Answer c

This patient is highly vulnerable and highly complex given the high catabolic state. The nursing characteristics of collaboration and clinical judgment are desired. Making expert judgments based on the whole picture and facilitating interdisciplinary practice will optimize the patient outcomes. The best initial consult would be for the registered dietician to be consulted to optimize the nutrition support therapy. Choices a, b, and d would not be initial consults for the highly catabolic patient.

REFERENCES

Annis, T. D. (2002). The Synergy Model in Practice: The Interdisciplinary Team Across the Continuum of Care. *Critical Care Nurse* 22(5): 76–79.

Curley, M. A.Q. (1998). Patient-Nurse Synergy: Optimizing Patients' Outcomes. *American Journal of Critical Care* 7(1): 64–72.
Collopy, K. S. (1999). The Synergy Model in Practice: Advanced Practice Nurses Guiding Families Through Systems. *Critical Care Nurse* 19(5): 80–5.

20. Answer b

The nurse characteristic of facilitator of learning is the most needed at this time. Choice a assumes that family members are all willing. Choice c does not incorporate clustering portions of procedures into learning sections. Teaching an entire procedure at once would not be optimal—and choice d is not correct. Facilitating education programs for patient's families begins with the needs assessment. Choice b would be a portion of the assessment that is the initial part of a teaching plan.

REFERENCES

Curley, M. A.Q. (1998). Patient-Nurse Synergy: Optimizing Patients' Outcomes. *American Journal of Critical Car,* 7(1): 64–72.
Collopy, K. S. (1999). The Synergy Model in Practice: Advanced Practice Nurses Guiding Families Through Systems. *Critical Care Nurse* 19(5): 80–5.

21. Answer c

The nurse characteristics of clinical inquiry and systems thinking are used to incorporate the best response for this issue. A description of clinical inquiry is that it communicates research results to nursing staff. In addition, systems thinking incorporates a variety of strategies, which may include applying research findings to meet the needs of patients. Knowing that the practice of administering boluses of liquids to liquefy secretions is not substantiated in the literature. The most appropriate response would be to discuss the research findings with the nursing peer.

REFERENCES

Curley, M. A.Q. (1998). Patient-Nurse Synergy: Optimizing Patients' Outcomes. *American Journal of Critical Care* 7(1): 64–72.
Schwenker, D., Ferrin, M. & Gift, A. G. (1998). Controversies in Critical Care: A Survey of Endotracheal Suctioning with Instillation of Normal Saline. Advanced Practice Nurses Guiding Families Through Systems. *Critical Care Nurse* 7(4): 255–260.

22. Answer c

The use of the nurse characteristics of clinical judgment and clinical inquiry would best meet the needs of the patient and family members at this time. In order to communicate results to the patient/family dyad at this time, and to continue to develop the plan of care, further information is needed. Asking open-ended questions would facilitate the continuance of conversation. Choices a, b, and d would only illicit a yes or no response.

REFERENCES

Curley, M. A.Q. (1998). Patient-Nurse Synergy: Optimizing Patients' Outcomes. *American Journal of Critical Care* 7(1): 64–72.
Collopy, K. S. (1999). The Synergy Model in Practice: Advanced Practice Nurses Guiding Families Through Systems. *Critical Care Nurse* 19(5): 80–5.

23. Answer b

The capacity of this patient to return to a restorative level of functioning is identified as moderate level because the patient is weak and unable to participate. Due to the criticism from the family members, the complexity of the patient/family dynamic would be identified as highly complex. The nurse characteristics needed at this time include advocacy/moral agency to ensure the rights of the patients and their families. In addition, a collaborative and caring environment would optimally promote patient outcomes; thus, choice b is needed to facilitate discussion of issues regarding patient care. Rotating the assignment or limiting visitation will not address the issue—and choice c is not correct.

REFERENCES

Curley, M. A.Q. (1998). Patient-Nurse Synergy: Optimizing Patients' Outcomes. *American Journal of Critical Care* 7(1): 64–72.
Mullen, J. E. (2002). The Synergy Model in Practice: The Synergy Model as a Framework for Nursing Rounds. *Critical Care Nurse* 22(6): 66–79.

24. Answer a

Knowing that the son desires to participate in care, it is important that the nurse as the facilitator of learning provides adequate opportunity for successful re-demonstration of learned skills. The best intervention for the next step is to provide opportunities for the son to practice the newly learned skill. Options b, c, and d will not provide for this intervention, thus would not be the appropriate next step.

REFERENCES

Curley, M. A.Q. (1998). Patient-Nurse Synergy: Optimizing Patients' Outcomes. *American Journal of Critical Care* 7(1): 64–72.

Collopy, K. S. (1999). The Synergy Model in Practice: Advanced Practice Nurses Guiding Families Through Systems. *Critical Care Nurse* 19(5): 80–5.

25. Answer a

The patient/family dyad is highly vulnerable and minimally stable given that they have not left the bedside for 5 days. The extent to which they engage in decision making is moderately limited given the expressed anger toward the health care team. Until further assessment is made to clarify the problem, teaching, and giving further information, choices b and d will not address the problem. Choice c is not the first intervention that should be incorporated. The nursing characteristics of advocacy/moral agency and caring practices will optimally assist to navigate the patient as the transition occurs along the health care continuum. The first step is to reassess and clarify the problem, and then the plan of care can be continued.

REFERENCES

Curley, M. A.Q. (1998). Patient-Nurse Synergy: Optimizing Patients' Outcomes. *American Journal of Critical Care* 7(1): 64–72.

Mullen, J. E. (2002). The Synergy Model in Practice: The Synergy Model as a Framework for Nursing Rounds. *Critical Care Nurse* 22(6): 66–79.

GLOSSARY

PATIENT CHARACTERISTICS

Complexity: The intricate entanglement of two or more systems, such as body, family, and therapies.

Participation in care: The extent to which the patient and family engage in aspects of care.

Participation in decision making: The extent to which the patient and family engage in decision making.

Predictability: A characteristic that allows one to expect certain events or a course of illness.

Resiliency: The capacity to return to a restorative level of functioning by using compensatory coping mechanisms.

Resource availability: The extent of resources that a patient, family, or community bring to a situation.

Stability: The ability to maintain a steady-state equilibrium.

Vulnerability: Susceptibility to actual or potential stressors that may adversely affect patient outcomes.

NURSE CHARACTERISTICS

Advocacy/moral agency: Working on another's behalf and representing the concerns of patients, families, and/or nursing staff and serving as a moral agent in identifying and resolving ethical and clinical concerns within or outside the clinical setting.

Caring practices: A constellation of nursing activities that creates a compassionate, supportive, and therapeutic environment with patients and staff. The aim is to promote comfort, heal, and prevent unnecessary suffering.

Clinical inquiry: The ongoing process of questioning and evaluating practice, providing informed practice, and creating practice changes through research utilization and experiential knowledge.

Clinical judgment: Clinical reasoning that includes clinical decision making, critical thinking, and a global grasp of the situation, as well as nursing skills required through a process of integrating formal and experiential knowledge.

Collaboration: Working with others, including physicians, families, and other health care providers in a way that promotes and encourages each person's contributions toward achieving optimal, realistic patient goals. Collaboration involves intradisciplinary and interdisciplinary work with colleagues.

Facilitator of learning: The ability to help patients, nursing staff, physicians, and other health care disciplines learn both formally and informally.

Response to diversity: The sensitivity to recognize, appreciate, and incorporate differences into the provision of care. Differences may include, but are not limited to, individuality, cultural differences, spiritual beliefs, gender, race, ethnicity, disability, family configuration, lifestyle, socioeconomic status, age, values, and alternative medicine involving patients' families and members of the health care team.

Systems thinking: A body of knowledge and tools that allows the nurse to manage whatever environmental and system resources exist for the patient, family, and staff within or across health care and nonhealth care systems.

INDEX